CREATIVE ARTS THERAPY CAREERS

Succeeding as a Creative Professional

EDITED BY SALLY BAILEY

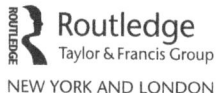
Routledge
Taylor & Francis Group

NEW YORK AND LONDON

First published 2022
by Routledge
605 Third Avenue, New York, NY 10158

and by Routledge
2 Park Square, Milton Park, Abingdon, Oxon, OX14 4RN

Routledge is an imprint of the Taylor & Francis Group, an informa business

Library of Congress Cataloging-in-Publication Data
Names: Bailey, Sally D., editor.
Title: Creative arts therapy careers / edited by Sally Bailey.
Description: New York, NY: Routledge, 2022. | Includes bibliographical references and index.
Identifiers: LCCN 2021017071 (print) | LCCN 2021017072 (ebook) | ISBN 9780367476526 (hardback) | ISBN 9780367476533 (paperback) | ISBN 9781003035664 (ebook)
Subjects: LCSH: Art therapy--Vocational guidance. | Arts--Therapeutic use.
Classification: LCC RC489.A7 C74 2022 (print) | LCC RC489.A7 (ebook) | DDC 616.89/1656023--dc23
LC record available at https://lccn.loc.gov/2021017071
LC ebook record available at https://lccn.loc.gov/2021017072

ISBN: 978-0-367-47652-6 (hbk)
ISBN: 978-0-367-47653-3 (pbk)
ISBN: 978-1-003-03566-4 (ebk)

DOI: 10.4324/9781003035664

Typeset in Adobe Garamond Pro and Avenir
by Deanta Global Publishing Services, Chennai, India

Dedicated to my drama therapy mentors who helped me learn the craft of the trade and who opened doors into the profession for me:

Janet Goodrich

Linda Gregoric Cook

Norman Fedder

Patricia Sternberg

CONTENTS

FOREWORD

Anna Weinstein

Creating a work of art is, by its very nature, a therapeutic practice. We create because we *must*. Not so much because we owe it to ourselves to make art but rather because, if we don't make art, those creative energies bubbling to the surface are bound to come out in some form – and we recognize that it'll likely be better for those spirits to emerge in art than in life!

We express our fears and hopes through our art. We process our losses, celebrate our good fortune, ponder our existence, imagine loves who might have been, mourn loves who once were.

We have gained something by the time we complete a work of art. If nothing else, a sense of calm. A bit of relief. That act of creating enabled us to put our thoughts and feelings into something outside of ourselves. It was, as it turns out, *therapeutic*.

Equally rewarding, of course, is the knowledge that by sharing our art, we might just provide some relief for our audience. We've all listened to music that has moved us to tears or inspired us to dance or skip or smile. We've watched films and read novels and studied paintings that seem to be speaking directly to us. And these works of art help us process the complexities of our own experiences and emotions. If that musician wrote those lyrics, it's proof she understands what we're going through! We memorize and recite the lyrics because it's therapeutic to do so.

And this is what creative arts therapists understand about the healing nature of art: Art and therapy are intrinsically connected.

I am honored and incredibly excited to share this volume with you. Sally Bailey has compiled a collection of insights from world-renowned creative arts therapists whose work in music therapy, drama therapy, dance therapy, expressive arts therapy, language arts therapy – and the many subcategories within each of these! – will open your mind to the myriad possibilities this field has to offer.

In these pages, you will find descriptions of how creative arts therapists developed their skills as therapists; where and how they trained under the guidance of mentors and licensed supervisors; how they learned to work with clients of all ages from a variety of backgrounds; how they created and marketed their own businesses; how they advocate for their clients; and how they have worked to stop the stigma of mental illness.

This is one of the most moving aspects of this volume, its focus on mental health. Whether you're just beginning to explore the possibilities in creative arts therapy or you're already working professionally in the field, I am certain you will be encouraged by the work so many of Sally's colleagues are doing to support people struggling with their mental health.

This recollection from Azizi Marshall, founder and CEO of the Center for Creative Arts Therapy in Downers Grover, Illinois, exemplifies the heart of all the essays and interviews in this volume:

> Growing up in a household of two artistic psychotherapist parents, I learned at an early age that people are beautifully complex. I was witness to how the arts could guide extremely troubled individuals and communities to a place of healing and growth. I observed my father transform his clients from people who hated life to people who loved themselves. It was not through traditional talk therapy, but through a therapeutic intervention called psychodrama: the marrying of psychotherapy and [theater].

I love Azizi's recollection about the origins of her interest in this work. It's a poignant reminder that no matter the type of artist we are, no matter where we are in the trajectory of our own life and work, when we combine our passion for the creative arts and our desire to be of service to others, opportunities for healing arise.

There is a spirit of generosity and kindness in the voices of every contributor in this volume. The stories and wisdom woven throughout the book are uplifting, encouraging, and enlightening, which is *exactly* my goal for every book in the PERFORM series.

A heartfelt thank you to Sally for the tremendous work she put into gathering and sharing these insights. What a gift to us all!

I hope you will find in these pages answers to your questions and inspiration for your own work and creative practice. Wishing you the very best.

Anna Weinstein is series editor of PERFORM: Succeeding as a creative professional.

ACKNOWLEDGMENTS

This book came about after I emailed Anna Weinstein, the series editor of *Perform: Succeeding as a Creative Professional*, to suggest that she include an essay in one of the future books about careers in creative arts therapy. What I didn't know was that Anna's sister was a music therapist, and so she knew how gratifying a career in the creative arts therapies could be. Instead of asking me to write an essay for a book, she offered to let me jump into editing an entire book that included information about all the creative arts therapies.

Deep gratitude goes to all the authors who contributed essays for this book. Each time I contacted one of them (some of them colleagues, and some people I had never met before), they responded with enthusiasm and said, "Why hasn't someone written a book like this before?" I responded, "Well, it's time now – would you like to be part of it?" And despite all of the bizarre events that happened in 2020, from the COVID-19 pandemic to the economic meltdown to horrific weather events to racial protests, all my essay writers came through. One author had a tree blown through the roof of his home and several caught the COVID virus (thankfully all recovered). We all survived! Even better, each essay arrived so well-written, that very few changes needed to made, making my job very easy.

Thanks to photographer Geri Kodey, who translated her color photos of Kevin Spencer teaching magic into black and white. The rest of the photos were translated to black and white my sister Sue Leo, who volunteered her graphic design skills so more photos could be included in the book.

Thanks also go to Lucia Accorsi, the editor at Routledge for the book series, who was always available to answer questions and help.

I always tell people that being a drama therapist is the best way to make a living. I think any of our authors would say the same about working as a creative art therapist in their field. We all hope that those of you who read this book, who love the arts, psychology, and service to others, will be inspired to join us in the work we love.

INTRODUCTION

Sally Bailey

The creative arts therapies have been around for many years, long before the first professional associations came into being. Many creative arts therapies trace their origins back to ancient Greek civilization and the philosophies of Aristotle. During the Roman Empire in the second century AD, Soranus, a physician who worked with people who were mentally ill, prescribed reading or seeing a comedy as an intervention for depression and a tragedy for mania (Cockerham, 2000). In the 1800s, music, art, and poetry were used alongside horticulture as tools by Dr. Benjamin Rush and other proponents of "moral therapy" to calm and rehabilitate patients in mental hospitals (Cockerham, 2000).

Occupational therapists used the arts in psychiatric hospitals in the first half of the twentieth century. Psychiatrists recognized that patients involved in the arts made quicker recoveries than patients who were not (Phillips, 1996). Dr. T. D. Noble, of Shepard-Pratt Institute, remarked in 1933 that drama was "a vehicle for both the discovery and expression of unconscious conflicts" (Phillips, 1996, p. 231). Moreover, he felt drama provided patients with a way to experiment with behavior, making them more flexible and open to change (Phillips, 1996). After each world war, when soldiers, who had what is now called Post Traumatic Syndrome Disorder, could not recover from their traumatic experiences on the battlefield through talk therapy, the creative arts therapies were

DOI: 10.4324/9781003035664-101

used to help them express themselves and heal. Through those successes, each of the creative art therapies grew as bona fide professions.

As the professionals who combined arts with psychotherapy began practicing, they banded together in professional associations to create educational standards, best practices, and codes of ethics. The first music therapy association (NAMT) was founded as a non-profit professional organization in 1950 (it is now the American Music Therapy Association – AMTA); the American Dance Therapy Association (ADTA) began in 1966; the American Art Therapy Association (AATA) was established in 1969; the North American Drama Therapy Association (NADTA) was incorporated in 1979; and the National Association for Poetry Therapy (NAPT) was formed in 1986. The International Expressive Art Therapy Association (IEATA) was founded in 1994 by creative art therapists who believed combining all the arts together is an even more effective therapeutic strategy. However, even with 50+ years in existence, the creative arts therapies still seem like a well-kept secret to most of the American public.

The purpose of this book is to introduce young people studying the arts in high school and college to the creative arts therapies, so they can begin to seriously consider a career as an art, music, dance/movement, drama, expressive arts, or poetry therapist. The book, like others in the *Perform* series, is made up of five chapters. The first, "Getting Started," begins with an essay that clarifies the differences among the many possible careers in the arts: from professional artist to educator to arts-in-health professional to creative arts therapist. This is followed by essays or interviews with four creative arts therapists about how they discovered their path to the creative arts therapies. Chapter One ends with a call for Black, Indigenous, and People of Color (BIPOC) students to consider becoming creative arts therapists (CATs) in order to provide role models who truly understand the cultural context of clients of similar backgrounds. Currently in creative arts therapies, as in all psychotherapy fields, there is a dearth of BIPOC therapists. We need more!

After graduating from high school or college, many in the visual and performing arts take jobs as waiters, secretaries, or administrators that temporarily pay the bills, while they attempt to do their art on the side. This can be exhausting, and, often, there is not much time in which to actually practice their craft. Often visual and performing artists only see limited choices before them: to become a professional artist, to teach their art, or to do something that has nothing to do with their art. However, there are more options than that.

How can you discern if a career in the creative arts is a good choice for you? There are many opportunities to practice your art in your community and to help others at the same time. Summer camps and afterschool or weekend programs are always looking for counselors and teachers who have genuine talents they can pass on to children or adults. Some programs focus on people who have physical, mental, emotional, or cognitive disabilities and struggle with aspects of day-to-day life. Others focus on children or youth-at-risk. Entertaining patients in hospitals or families at libraries through puppet shows is a wonderful way to provide enjoyment, as well as educational and therapeutic experiences for community members. There may be refugees or immigrants in your community who need to learn new skills, including language and cultural awareness, in order to become employable. The same is true of community members who are homeless, recovering from mental illnesses, or unemployed. Older adults need to find new connections with others after losing family members and friends or after developing physical or mental impairments that narrow their options for recreational and social engagement. Working in jobs like these as a volunteer or paid employee allows a young artist to test out their aptitude for working with others and decide whether the creative arts therapies would be a viable and positive option as a career.

The second chapter, "Sticking it out," contains essays by professors who teach creative art therapies at different universities. All have spent time practicing as CATs within their modality before transitioning to training the next generation of CATs. Requirements for curricula for each creative art therapy are set by the professional organization of each art modality. The authors in this section share the courses, internships, and other learning opportunities that comprise the degree programs in their fields. While universities follow association guidelines, each program is unique in their faculty, philosophies, and teaching styles. More information on education and approved university programs in each creative art modality are available on the websites of each professional organization.

Chapter three, "Finding Success," provides examples of what starting a career as a creative arts therapist might entail. The authors in this section explain what an employer is looking for in a new hire, the importance of supervision, how to transition from working with one population of clients to another, and the importance of connecting with fellow CATs.

Chapter four is entitled "Getting Ahead." Once an early career CAT has earned a specific number of professional hours (each discipline requires a different amount), they are able to apply for registry, the national credential in their art modality. Some organizations require applications with letters of recommendations and essays; others require tests, demonstrations, or written case studies. As experience is gained, CATs need continuing education and attend conferences in order to keep their skills sharp and learn about new discoveries in their field. As they mature, they may decide to take on management or supervisory responsibilities at their job, branch out to work with new populations of clients, begin to present at conferences, write about their work in books, publish research articles in professional journals, or become consultants. Some practitioners fall in love with another creative art modality and become credentialed in more than one. Any of these activities can lead to more income opportunities, additional respect, and the ability to guide beginners and give back to their field.

The final chapter, "Starting Again," covers other opportunities that may be offered to CATs. Some practitioners may be asked to create an organization to offer more comprehensive services to their clients. This happened to Loretta Gallo-Lopez when parents of her clients asked that she start Focus Academy. Others create centers where a group of creative arts therapists can practice together as Azizi Marshall did with the Center for Creative Arts Therapy in Downer's Grove, Illinois. Sometimes opportunities exist to incorporate a whole new set of techniques into their work, as Kevin Spencer describes in "Magic Therapy." CATs may take on advocating with government offices to expand access to therapy for their clients as Michelle Yadon and Tracena Marie did in Indiana, or they might work toward creating licensure for creative arts therapists in their state as the New Jersey Task Force on Drama Therapy and Dance/Movement Therapy did. Advocacy can also mean empowering clients to speak up about their experiences as they were able to do through Village Playback Theatre's tour to break down the stigma of mental illness.

Creative arts therapists love their jobs. We don't want our fields to be a secret. We wish more young artists knew that a career in the creative arts therapies would offer them a wonderful, fulfilling life. We hope that this book gets you excited about looking further into the creative arts therapies as your future profession.

References

Cockerham, W. C. (2000). *Sociology of mental disorder.* (5th ed.). Hoboken, NJ: Prentice-Hall.

Phillip, M. E. (1996). The use of drama and puppetry in occupational therapy in the 1920's and 1930's. *The American Journal of Occupational Therapy, 50*(3), 229–233.

CHAPTER 1

GETTING STARTED

Sally Bailey, Laura Wood, Kareen King,
Teri Holmberg, Mariah Meyer LeFeber,
Sarah Edwards, and Denise Boston

A Preview of Coming Attractions: Discovering the Creative Arts Therapies

As mentioned in the Introduction, Chapter One: Getting Started shares stories of how several young artists discovered the creative arts therapies and realized that they offered an exciting and fulfilling way to make a living. Laura Wood begins by offering an essay that overviews careers in the arts: artist, art educator, artist in healthcare, and creative arts therapist. She shares how she found drama therapy and made the transition from theater to therapy.

Next Kareen King, another drama therapist, shares how she had included all the arts – visual, music, and performing arts through puppetry and educational puppet plays – in her work in her husband's ministry and as a freelance puppeteer. When she discovered there was a drama therapy training program near her, even though she had little formal training in theater, she decided to give it a try to expand her abilities. She found she had been a theater person all along and thrived in the drama therapy world.

Teri Holmberg started as a music educator in the public schools and quickly realized that a master's degree in music therapy would make her more effective

DOI: 10.4324/9781003035664-1

with the students she was teaching. As she says, "music therapy interventions … served as a vehicle for removing barriers to students' ability to demonstrate skills they already had."

Sarah Edwards trained in theater, and, while working as a freelance theater educator in Tennessee, discovered how effective drama was for job skills training for people with disabilities. She realized she loved working with this population of people but felt she needed more training to do it ethically and responsibly. Following the suggestion of an undergraduate professor, she got her master's in drama therapy. Now she is back at Friends Life making a difference in people's lives.

Mariah Meyer LeFeber double-majored in dance and psychology because, while psychology seemed like an interesting and proper subject to study as an undergraduate, she couldn't let go of her love of dance. Later she realized she could put the two disciplines together to integrate her passions and help others. This has allowed her to experience a career that gives her joy and allows her to share that joy with her clients.

Finally, Denise Boston writes about the need in the profession of therapy in general, and the creative arts therapies specifically, for therapists who come from and represent marginalized communities. Clients from those communities, whether Black, Indigenous, or People of Color (BIPOC), Lesbian, Gay, Bisexual, Transgender, Queer, Intersex, or Asexual (LGBTQIA+), or persons with disabilities, need to have the option of working with professionals who look like them and share their experiences. This does not mean that BIPOC clients should only go to BIPOC therapists and white clients should only go to white therapists; it means clients should have the option of choosing a therapist who has experienced the same societal struggles they have had.

TAPESTRY OF TRANSFORMATION: PATHWAYS IN THE ARTS PROFESSIONS

▶ by Laura L. Wood

Laura L. Wood, PhD, RDT–BCT, LMHC, CCLS is an associate professor at Lesley University, teaching in their Clinical Mental Health Counseling and Expressive Therapy Program. She is a licensed mental health counselor (LMHC), registered drama therapist/board-certified trainer (RDT–BCT), and a certified child life specialist (CCLS). Dr. Wood specializes in the treatment of eating disorders, trauma, dissociation, and recovery with different populations. She publishes and lectures on these areas nationally and internationally.

An Overview of Careers in the Arts

We are increasingly understanding the transformative benefits of the arts, as contemporary research finds profound scientific evidence of the arts' powerful effects on the brain and body (Clift & Camic, 2016). Given this, there is a growing interest in the application of the arts to many different arenas: social, educational, medical, behavioral, and emotional. Thus, there are more opportunities than ever before to find a meaningful career in the field of the arts and healing.

There are many different pathways to consider when thinking about a career in the domain of arts and transformation. Having taught at the undergraduate and graduate level, being connected to local high school Thespian chapters, and taking a few circuitous steps in the arts myself, I have had the opportunity to encounter myriad misconceptions about the different professions in the creative arts and what they encompass. This essay will clarify some of the different professions that involve the arts and transformation, their education requirements, and, I hope, help you get headed in the right direction.

It can be helpful to think of the arts as threads that each get interwoven into society to create a beautiful tapestry that enriches the human spirit, mind, and

CAREERS IN THE ARTS

Fine Arts	Arts in Education	Recreational Arts	Creative Arts Therapies	Arts in Health
Fine Artist (pottery, painting, mixed media, sculpture, photography, graphic design, etc.)	Kindergarten through 12th grade educator of an arts discipline (art teacher, etc.)	Teaching artist (for example in an after-school, community, or religious program)	Art Therapist	Teaching artist who works in a hospital program Architect
Professional writer (novel, short story, poetry, editor, etc.)	Undergraduate, Master, or Doctoral level educator of the arts disciplines	Community Theater	Poetry Therapist Bibliotherapist	Teaching artist who works in a hospital program
Actor/Performer (stage, television, film, voice over, director, etc.)	Museum educator or curator	Local arts programming (summer camp, YMCA, etc.)	Drama Therapist	Hospital Social Worker
Musician (opera singer, orchestra or band member, conductor etc.)	Music teacher, Band director.		Music Therapist	Music Thanatology
Dancer (ballet, modern, folk, choreographer, etc.)	Dance teacher	Community Theatre Choreographer	Dance/ Movement Therapist	
Combined Arts			Expressive Arts Therapist	

Careers in the Arts

Figure 1.1 Careers in the arts.

body. Figure 1.1 helps to visualize some of the various arts professions and a few of the ways that the arts can be used. It is by no means comprehensive. There are also administrators, boards, and other roles that help drive these professions, but these are some core professions that link to the arts directly.

Fine arts

The fine arts include drama, music, art, dance, and poetry/literature. Individuals on this pathway most often begin with the intention of becoming a professional actor, artist, dancer, or writer. People called to this career have often been profoundly impacted by the arts and possess a high degree of skill, talent, and innovation. They often aspire to use their craft to touch the lives of others, to create beauty, or change in the world at large (Oakley, Speary, & Pratt, 2008). Although not a requirement, many individuals, hoping for a career as a professional artist, attend a four-year undergraduate degree program that provides both a broad education in their chosen discipline as well as supports students in specializing in a specific technique or style. For example, if you choose to major in theater in your undergraduate studies, you will likely receive a broad education that will introduce you to many aspects of working in the theater, for example, acting, directing, design, and stage management. You will also likely specialize in one of these areas – like acting. And within that specialization, you may even get more specific training, such as focusing on acting for film and television, or musical theater, or a specific approach to acting such as the Stanislavsky or Meisner technique (Hodge, 2010).

The unfortunate joke that is often made to undergraduates (or those considering embarking on this pathway) is to prepare to wait tables or to have a backup plan. Many times, the general public doesn't understand that whether or not you decide to pursue your craft in the traditional sense, there are many other routes to a creative life that often require, or are strongly enhanced by, a degree in the fine arts. Additionally, sometimes people pursue their craft and end up growing or changing but still desire to apply the arts in their career in other ways. Others decide to deepen their craft and pursue a master's degree in their specialty area. Whichever way is chosen, a solid foundation in the arts provides many pathways.

Salary ranges for professional artists are vast and often skewed by those who are top earners in their craft versus those who are not. Each discipline has its own union or organization that individuals can qualify for, which will help them better understand salary options and provide community support. While this list is not comprehensive, it provides a good starting point for those who want to learn more (Figure 1.2).

Arts in education

Arts in education includes both being an *educator in the arts* or a *teaching artist*. An *educator in the arts* teaches their craft or the history of their craft in an educational curriculum, including kindergarten through twelfth grade and the collegiate level. *Educators in the arts* typically have a minimum of a bachelor's degree, usually in their specialty area, as well as a teaching certificate. Many go on to get a master's degree in teaching within their art's discipline, which will refine their arts practice and have special emphasis on pedagogy, theories of

Arts Discipline	Example of an organizing body or union
Theater Artists	Actors Equity (https://www.actorsequity.org/) Screen Actors' Guild/American Federation of Television and Radio Artists (https://www.sagaftra.org)
Orchestral Musicians	American Federation of Musicians (https://www.afm.org)
Operatic, Choral, and Dance Heritage	American Guild of Musical Artists (https://www.musicalartists.org)
Fine Artists	Each discipline tends to have its own organizing body, for example: Oil Painters of America (https://www.oilpaintersofamerica.com/index.cfm) Portrait Society of America (https://www.portraitsociety.org)
Professional Writers	National Writers Union (https://nwu.org)

Organizing Bodies or Unions for Professional Artists

Figure 1.2 Organizing bodies and unions for professional artists.

learning, development, and curriculum planning. Furthermore, many who go on to get master's degrees in their specialty areas will also specialize in an age group (i.e., elementary arts education, arts in special education, etc.).

The overall role and function of *educators in the arts* is to deliver developmentally appropriate skills in their discipline to enrich students' knowledge and growth. And likely, if you are reading this book, you know it goes well beyond that. *Educators in the arts* often feel called to bring inspiration to students through their discipline, creating community and instilling the deep value that arts play in our culture and society (Karkou & Glasman, 2004). *Educators in the arts* can be generalists and work with a wide range of students in terms of age, ability, and skill level, or they can work in highly specialized areas, such as at a magnet arts schools or at the college level training pre-professionals. *Educators in the arts* may also partner with other academics, such as history, English, or science teachers, to use the arts to help approach material and add dimension to learning (Chapell et al., 2007). They typically work full-time in recognized educational institutions.

The O*Net Resource Center is a leading source for occupational salaries (https://www.onetcenter.org). At the time of this writing, the median salary for *educators in the arts* is US$69,530 with the range depending on geographic location and type of employment institution. O*Net also has a search function for individuals to look at regional differences. At the collegiate level, the starting salary for an assistant professor with an advanced degree (MFA or PhD) was reported by the American Association of University Professors to be US$75,000 in 2018 (www.aaup.org). There are many organizing bodies for *educators in the arts*, with each discipline having their own subgroups with more comprehensive information. Additionally, information can be found at conferences and in journals that support the profession.

Teaching artists are those who use their craft to support educational or community goals (Booth, 2003). They often hold a strong primary identity as an artist and are passionate about sharing their work and craft with communities to make both small and large changes (www.teachingartistsguild.org). *Teaching artists* may or may not have a degree in their specialty area. There is strong debate over whether being a *teaching artist* is a formal profession or a practice (Booth, 2003). Many of the jobs available for *teaching artists* have varying degrees of educational requirements, but focus on mastery of one's craft, a strong personal portfolio in one's discipline, and a proven track record of being able to work with groups of people. *Teaching artist* jobs range widely in availability, time frame, and salary. Some institutions hire *teaching artists* to work on a per-diem (by the day) basis, other positions are grant-funded for a specific project or period of time, while others are only an hour or two a week at an institution. The range of how, where, and with whom teaching artists work is as broad as communities themselves. *Teaching artists* might work professionally as an artist and teach in a community setting, such as a watercolor class at a senior center once a week. Others are devoted to full-time work solely as *teaching artists*, like being hired to lead a community-based social justice poetry project.

Teaching artist salaries are harder to pin down than other arts professions due to the transient nature of the work and reliance of the economy for grant-funded positions. However, one popular organizing body, the Teaching Artist Guild (https://teachingartistsguild.org), provides a geographical calculator to support teaching artists in calculating fair wages. Payscale.com reported in 2019 that *teaching artists'* median hourly salary in the USA was US$20.52 an hour. This website is a wonderful resource to support learning more about the opportunities and the challenges of committing to a career as a *teaching artist*.

Arts-in-health

The field of arts-in-health, sometimes termed arts-in-medicine, is an umbrella term that encompasses professions invested in using the power of the arts to enhance health and well-being in diverse institutional health care settings. These arts experiences can either be passive or participatory (NOAH, 2017). *Arts-in-health professionals* are made up of professional artists, artist consultants, teaching artists, creative arts therapists, arts educators, architects, child life specialists, landscape architects, and healthcare arts administrators, each with their unique function in a larger hospital system that subscribes to a lens of the healing value of the arts. An *artist-in-healthcare, artist-in-residence,* or *arts practitioner* usually has a formal background in arts training and provides arts experiences to help shape the atmosphere of the health care setting. For example, an *artist-in-healthcare* might provide live music in the hospital lobby, be commissioned to create a meaningful mural in the intake area or conduct an arts-based project with those in a waiting area. *Artists-in-healthcare* work to create *therapeutic* environments using the arts but do not conduct therapy and are not licensed or credentialed professionals. *Artists-in-health* "differ from those associated with the six distinct creative arts therapies – that is, professionals who are designated as therapists, distinguished by legally defensible scopes of practice and certification/licensure" (NOAH, 2017, p. 23) which we will explore further in the next section.

The organizing body for this profession is the National Organization for Arts in Health (NOAH). In 2018, NOAH released their first code of ethics for *arts-in-health professionals* and reported that in the forthcoming years they will be moving towards creating a credential. It is unclear at the time of this publication who the credential will be targeting, but it could be a general credential intended for all who work as *arts-in-health professionals*, or it may be specifically for artists working as an *artist-in-healthcare* in order to provide them with a scope of practice, ethical framework, and shared knowledge base.

There are some emerging programs (both formal degree programs and advanced certificates) in the field of arts-in-health/medicine; however, they vastly range in their coursework offerings and length of training, depending on area of focus. Curricula tend to include courses designed to support students in examining and practicing the use of arts related to community wellness, and helping students gain knowledge and skills in understanding public health and policy.

Additionally, persons who might be part of an *arts-in-healthcare team* (architects, creative arts therapists, hospital administrators, etc.) will need to come to the table with a specific degree in their profession and may work to adopt or support an arts-in-healthcare/medicine framework without formal arts-in-medicine training. Therefore, pursuing training as an *arts-in-healthcare professional* would be focused toward persons who have a desire to run, coordinate, or promote arts-in-medicine programs and make meaningful change in public health policy.

Due to the wide range of jobs in the arts-in-health field, there is no median salary available at the time of publication. However, *artists-in-healthcare* often come from a *teaching artist* background and could expect to make similar salaries to *teaching artists'* rates in the area. Other professionals, who may work as part of an arts-in-healthcare team, could expect salaries commensurate with experience and on par with similar jobs in their respective professions.

Creative arts therapies

The *creative arts therapies* comprise a distinct professional group made up of highly trained individuals, who specialize in the use of their chosen art form, to help individuals, groups, and communities make meaningful psychological, behavioral, physical, and emotional change. There are five distinct types of creative arts therapies: drama therapy, music therapy, art therapy, dance/movement therapy, and poetry therapy (Malchiodi, 2020). Although these five professions all belong to one overarching organization, The National Coalition of Creative Arts Therapies (NCCATA), they each have their own regulating bodies that outline the specific educational, ethical, and extensive clinical experience requirements needed to practice. *Creative arts therapists* are both artists and clinical practitioners and must demonstrate mastery in both areas. Additionally, many *creative arts therapists* hold mental health licenses in their states of practice.

Creative arts therapists work in a wide range of settings including, but not limited to:

> adult day treatment centers, community mental health centers, community residences and halfway houses, correctional and forensic facilities, disaster relief centers, drug and alcohol programs, early intervention programs, general hospitals, home health agencies, hospices, neonatal nurseries, nursing homes, outpatient clinics, psychiatric units and hospitals, rehabilitative facilities, senior centers, schools, and wellness centers
>
> *(NOAH, 2017, p. 23).*

Some may also work in private practices, corporate companies, religious, or social justice-based community organizations.

Many individuals come to the creative arts therapies because they themselves have experienced or witnessed firsthand the inherent healing or transformative nature of the arts and seek to continue to use the arts in the helping professions.

In addition, they recognize the need for advanced training to ensure ethical practice.

Starting Out

For example, I spent most of my childhood acting. I took my first drama class when I was six years old. My mother was exhausted by my outgoing personality and wanted to channel her daughter's "ham" energy. Her instinct was spot on, and theater became an instant outlet for me. I no longer felt weird or different but with "my people." Furthermore, during my childhood, my family moved to a different state every three to four years. What I loved was that while the place I was living in looked different, the theater did not. Shows always had the same structure, theater kids were still unique and weird and welcoming, and the rituals of putting on a show were the same. Since I was a pretty good kid, a rule follower, and an overachiever, what I liked about theater was that I could "play" someone else. I could be a villain or a monster, and then leave the role behind.

When I went to college, I decided to study acting and went on to perform professionally. While I really enjoyed it, I also was influenced by living through 9/11 in New York City and witnessed the healing power that deep listening and the arts provided to people to help them cope with tragedy. While auditioning, I was also working part-time as a medical interpreter in American Sign Language for the Deaf and Hard community and running a summer arts camp on the west side of Manhattan. I loved the performing side of the work of being an actor, but I did not love the self-promotion and marketing that was required. I also did not want to leave the teaching/helping roles that I was running in summer camp and working as an interpreter. I became passionate about figuring out how I could combine all my interests and my love of helping people through the arts. That's when I realized I had created a new field: theater therapy! When I went to the library (Google wasn't around quite yet!), I found that I had, in fact, *not* created a new profession – it already existed. It was called drama therapy and was part of the Creative Arts Therapies. I learned that a drama therapist supports a person in taking on new roles in dramatic reality and practicing new ways of being, which then helps them apply that to their life at large (Landy, 1994). This was exactly what I loved about theater! I could try on new roles and then learn how to own those aspects in my life outside of the theater, which then gave me more options, spontaneity, freedom, and flexibility in the world. I no longer had to be one dimensional; I could tolerate contradictory feelings and ways of being in the world. Through drama therapy and theater, I realized, as Walt Whitman (1904) noted, "I am large, I contain multitudes."

Education in Creative Arts Therapies

While coursework varies for each profession, most creative arts therapy degrees are 60 credit-hour master's programs. Coursework often includes specialized training in assessment, diagnosis, theory, practice, refining one's craft, human development, diversity, equity, and inclusion, helping skills, group theory, research and evaluation, and the unique application of the arts specialty area to supporting change.

According to the US Bureau of Labor Statistics (www.bls.org) in 2018, depending on one's specialty area, the starting salary ranges from $41,000 to $51,000 for *creative arts therapists* who also held a state mental health counseling license. Salary increases commensurate with experience and leadership positions within the field of creative arts therapies.

Figure 1.3 presents different national associations in the creative arts therapies and each of their unique requirements.

Expressive therapy
Although the profession of expressive arts therapies is not a part of NCCATA, it is often considered to be part of the creative arts therapy profession. *Expressive art therapists* are trained more broadly in the application of more than one art and have a special focus on the way the different arts interplay with one another to help clients and communities making meaningful psychological and behavioral changes (Knill et al., 2005).

The regulating body for the field of *expressive arts therapists*, the International Expressive Arts Therapy Association (IEATA), prepares individuals to become a Registered Expressive Arts Therapist (REAT). The training to become a REAT includes comprehensive coursework and clinical training as well as certification requirements that have similarities to those of creative arts therapies. Both master's level training and certificate programs exist across the globe. Additionally, "IEATA is also currently the only professional association that acknowledges artists, educators, and consultants and offers a separate registration process for individuals in these categories" (NOAH, 2017, p. 22). *Expressive arts therapists* can expect to earn a similar salary to creative arts therapists if they also hold a mental health license. For more information see: https://www.ieata.org.

National associations of creative arts therapies and their unique requirements.					
	Music Therapy	Art Therapy	Dance Therapy	Drama Therapy	Poetry Therapy
National Association	American Music Therapy Association (AMTA)	American Art Therapy Association (AATA)	American Dance Therapy Association (ADTA)	North American Drama Therapy Association (NADTA)	The National Association for Poetry Therapy (NAPT)
Minimum Education Level Required to Practice	Bachelor's	Master's	Master's	Master's	Bachelor's + Master's
Education Levels Offered	Bachelor's, Master's, Doctorate	Bachelor's, Master's, Doctorate	Master's, Doctorate	Master's, Doctorate	N/A
Minimum Credentials or Professional Designations Required to Practice	Music Therapist – Board Certified (MT-BC) Exam required.	Registered Art Therapist (ATR)	Registered Dance/Movement Therapist (R-DMT)	Registered Drama Therapist (RDT)	Certified Applied Poetry Facilitator (CAPF) Bachelor's level
Credentialing Agency	Certification Board for Music Therapists (CBMT)	Art Therapy Credentials Board, Inc. (ATCB)	Dance/Movement Therapy Certification Board (DMTCB)	NADTA	The Int'l Federation for Biblio-Poetry Therapy (IFB/PT)
Training Required for Credentials	1200 hrs. supervised clinical training, including practicum and internship	700 hrs. supervised practicum during Master's, 1000 paid clinical hrs. post-graduate w/ 100 hrs. supervision (in most states)	200 hrs. supervised fieldwork, 700 hrs. practicum w/ 70 hrs. supervision during Master's	800 hrs. supervised practicum during master's w/ at least 30 hrs. supervision 1500 paid clinical hrs. post-graduate	CAPF + CPT 440 hrs. training/ supervision RPT 975 hrs. training/ supervision
Advanced Credentials and/or Professional Designation/ Specialized Training Certificates	Fellow-Guided Imagery and Music Hospice and Palliative Care Music Therapy Neonatal Intensive Care Unit Music Therapist. Neurologic Music Therapist Nordoff-Robbins Music Therapist	Registered Art Therapist – Board Certified (ATR-BC) Exam required.	Board Certified Dance/Movement Therapist (BC-DMT) 3640 paid hrs. + Exam required.	Registered Drama Therapist/ Board Certified Trainer (RDT/BCT) 5 yrs. experience as RDT + evaluation by Board of Examiners.	Certified Poetry Therapist (CPT) Registered Poetry Therapist (RPT) Master's + Licensure in a mental health field required.
Code of Professional Practice/ Ethics	Yes	Yes	Yes	Yes	Yes
Legally Defensible Scope of Practice	Yes	Yes	Yes	Yes	Yes
Continuing Education Required	100 CEUs every 5 years for MT-BC	100 CEUs every 5 years ATR-BC only	100 CEUs every 5 years BC-DMT only	RDT: 30 CEUs every 2 yrs. BCT: BCT training	20 CEUs every 2 yrs.
State Licensure Required	In several states: www.cbmt.org for more info	In several states contact: info@arttherapy.org for more info	In several states Contact: info@adta.org for more info	NY and NJ	N/A

Chart from www.thenoah.net

Figure 1.3 National associations of creative arts therapies and their unique requirements.

Conclusion

I hope you are beginning to see there are many options open to using the arts to create profound change in both formal and informal ways. Most importantly, do your research before you head into your next direction. Mentorship has been shown to be critical in supporting those in the creative arts professions (Frydman et al., 2018). Find a person who is working in the profession to connect with, take an introductory course, or find out if it would be appropriate to attend a professional conference. Any of these will likely enrich your understanding of the profession and help crystalise your next steps. As Pablo Picasso reminds us, "Art washes away from the soul the dust of everyday life." So, no matter how you choose to work with the arts (or support them), they undoubtedly help us transcend, heal, and grow and are a noble profession to be part of.

References

Booth, E. (2003). Seeking definition: What is a teaching artist? *Teaching Artist Journal, 1*(1), 5–12.

Chappell, K., Slade, C., Greenwood, M., & Craft, A. (2007). CREAT-IT: A new pedagogical framework for partnering the arts and science in science education. *Research in Science Education*.

Clift, S., & Camic, P. M. (Eds.). (2016). *Oxford textbook of creative arts, health, and wellbeing: International perspectives on practice, policy and research*. Oxford University Press.

Frydman, J. S., Segall, J., & Wood, L. L. (2018). Themes of career advancement among North American drama therapists: A secondary qualitative analysis. *Drama Therapy Review, 4*(2), 271–286.

Hodge, A. (2010). *Actor training*. Routledge.

Karkou, V., & Glasman, J. (2004). Arts, education and society: The role of the arts in promoting the emotional wellbeing and social inclusion of young people. *Support for Learning, 19*(2), 57–65.

Knill, P. J., Levine, E. G., & Levine, S. K. (2005). *Principles and practice of expressive arts therapy: Toward a therapeutic aesthetics*. Jessica Kingsley Publishers.

Landy, R. J. (1994).*Drama therapy: Concepts and practices*. Charles C. Thomas Publisher.

Malchiodi, C. A. (2020). *Trauma and expressive arts therapy: Brain, body, and imagination in the healing process*. Guilford Press.

National Organization for the Arts in Health (2017). *Arts, health, and well-being in America*. San Diego, CA: Author. Retrieved from www.https://thenoah.net/noah-publications/

Oakley, K., Sperry, B., & Pratt, A. C. (2008). *The art of innovation: How fine arts graduates contribute to innovation*.

Whitman, W. (1904). *Song of Myself*... Done into print by the Roycrofters.

FINDING MY PATH BY FOLLOWING MY TALENTS AND STRENGTHS

▶ An Interview With Kareen King

Kareen King, MA, RDT is a registered drama therapist from Lawrence, Kansas. She uses music, movement, storytelling, improvisational theatre, and poetry with older adults in long-term care. She did not discover the creative arts therapies until she was in her forties, but she had been developing her artistic skills, imagination, and talents her whole life.

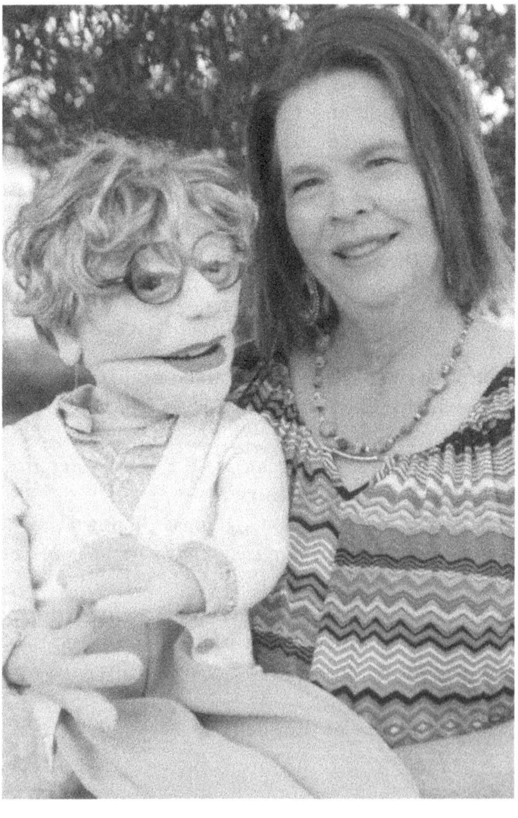

Figure 1.4 Drama Therapist Kareen King and her therapeutic puppet, Emilou.

You've always been involved in music. Did you study music growing up?

Yes! I took piano lessons from the age of six, and I learned how to sight-read but discovered I was better at playing by ear. So, I can do both. I took guitar lessons as a senior in high school, and I also play the clarinet. At 19, I realized I could write songs and have written over 500 songs so far.

What did you major in and what was your vision of your career when you left undergraduate school?

I went to four colleges and changed my major a few times. I had about 30 credit hours in music; I took courses in classical guitar, music and aural theory, music composition, voice, choral directing, and music for the elementary teacher. I decided I wanted to be an elementary school teacher, but then I realized I would have had to go to school for two more years to get a teaching degree beyond the four I'd already completed, and I wanted to graduate, so I ended up majoring in general studies and graduated with a total of 182 credit hours.

At the time I graduated I knew I had an interest in the arts and performance, but besides the music courses I'd taken, I had little training in the other arts. When my husband and I were first married, we were youth pastors and became interested in clowning. Since I was a seamstress, I sewed clown outfits for both of us. My husband learned to juggle, and we started doing ministry outreach using clowning to connect with children.

How else did you put your talents to work?

At 12, my parents gave me a puppet stage and that's when I learned that I could make character voices. Maybe that's when I became interested in performing. When I was a freshman at K-State, I took a free puppet-making workshop from a lady named Irma Kientz. I loved puppets, so I had to do that. Irma taught us to make moveable mouth puppets and gave us a free pattern. So, I just started making puppets.

I really got into puppets when my husband was an associate pastor at a church in Burlingame, Kansas. We started creating puppets for the children's ministry. We made little skits with puppets about kids who were different and who were bullied. I've always been an advocate for the downtrodden and overlooked.

Then as a young mother, I discovered that the local library had a summer reading program. That year the Wizard of Oz was the theme. So, I made puppets for the theme and volunteered to perform for them. Then I found out that The Northeast Kansas Library System had a conference once a year at which potential entertainers could audition for all the libraries across Kansas. The theme that year was *Paws and Claws*, about taking care of pets, so I auditioned with an original song called "How I Wish My Mom Would Let Me Have a Python for a Pet." That audition led to bookings in libraries all over northeast Kansas. After that, I created a new puppet musical each year based on the annual summer reading program theme. Jeff, my husband, made a new stage for me out of PVC pipe, and I sewed the curtains. I wrote the scripts and the songs. We also started doing grade school assemblies. I also produced professional recordings for two of the shows in which the music and voices were recorded. Then, as puppeteers, we only had to manipulate the puppets.

You told me that some of those shows were educational as well as fun.

My father was a psychiatrist, so I always had an interest in psychology. And there was my interest in being an educator and a mother. So, in addition to being musicals, the puppet shows ended up dealing a lot with helping kids understand and handle emotions. Inspired by the concept in the film *The Three Faces of Eve*, I created a puppet show called "The Three Faces of Stevie." One puppet was the regular Stevie, and then there was a red version of him that came up when he was angry, and a green version that came up when he was envious, and a yellow one when he was happy.

One of the shows for which I made a professional recording was called *Once There was a Bottle* about recycling and the environment. It was a huge hit. Every single puppet was made out of throwaway objects. The story followed a bottle that was thrown in the trash and then tossed into a pond, where the fish swallowed him, and it went on from there. Bottle puppets are the cutest puppets, and they are durable. I still have them – they've lasted a long time!

My last puppet musical, "The Globemeisters Meet Kansas!" was created in 1998 and was performed with my final puppet musical professional recording.

How did you discover drama therapy?

I never had any theatre background or was even in a play in school, with the exception of being a tree in the eighth grade, but I ended up being hired to teach a class called Theatre Appreciation at Allen County Community

College. In order to stay a step ahead of the students, I had a lot of catching up to do. So that first semester, I served as the accompanist for two musicals at two different theatres so I could observe the directors, did a documentary of a play, took a community acting class in Emporia, and took a comedy improv class in Topeka.

Students really liked the class, and I got good evaluations. The administration wanted me to teach public speaking, but they said I could only do so providing I started working on a master's degree. I liked that idea and thought, "What would I do?" My husband was studying to be a Marriage and Family Therapist at that point. We went to a Marriage and Family Conference in Nashville, and it was there that I spotted a brochure about the drama therapy program at Kansas State University. I knew in that moment it was something I'd like to explore.

Did your drama therapy career go in the direction you expected it to?

Absolutely not. In my drama therapy training, I interned with a lot of different populations, but I didn't know what I wanted to do, and I needed to get my professional hours somewhere after I graduated. I had only one community connection outside of the drama therapy program and our church, and that was the nursing home administrator at Brookside Retirement Community in Overbrook, Kansas (who I met because my husband did Bible studies for the residents at a previous nursing home in Osage City). I gave him a call and said, "Scott, I need to get my professional hours for drama therapy. Could I come in and do a drama therapy group with your residents once a week?" And he said, "How about a job?" So, I went in for an interview, and he hired me to be their full-time activity director.

I remember saying I didn't want to work with elders; I was sure about that! But I remember my major professor saying to me, "Give it a year so you can get enough hours to earn your registry." So, I said yes to the job, and then I ended up falling in love with the residents within the first week. I started writing songs that captured their life stories. I'd share the songs with them, their family, and staff. My boss supported me in having an album recorded of the songs. All the songs were about people who had been overlooked – who had dementia, were dying, residents who had no visitors, who wanted to go home, but couldn't.

A lot of people think I am a music therapist because I do so much with music. I also go weekly to a memory care home where I do music with them.

In a later chapter we will hear stories about the different directions that creative arts therapies careers have taken. I know your career has careened (no pun intended) in a number of different directions after your first job. Would you talk a little about that?

After several years, one of my coworkers at Overbrook asked if I would to do a concert of the songs I'd written about the residents for a luncheon for social workers. So, I did and told stories about the people who had inspired the songs and what they had taught me. The next day I got a call from the Kansas Healthcare Association's Director of Education asking me to be the keynote for their annual state conference. She said she'd just had three phone calls about the conference that I'd done the day before from people asking for me. At that point I was so naïve I didn't know what a keynote was. That keynote was the beginning of a 10-year run of doing keynotes and workshops for long-term care associations across the country.

I left my job as an activity director, and, except for one year when I took time to launch my own business, The Golden Experience (see www.thegoldenexperience.com), I've stayed in the trenches working with residents. After that one year I was asked to come back once a week to hold what I call Kareen's Kettle, a creative enrichment group that I facilitate for various groups of residents at two care communities. I try as hard as I can to engage everyone who comes to my programs. Everyone sits in a semi-circle, does warms-ups with me, sings fun songs, and explores a topic or theme through a variety of activities that support that theme. I have created well over 200 fully fleshed out creative engagement programs (Some were published in my book *"Engage! 28 Enrichment Experiences for Older Adults*, ArtAge Publications, 2014). For me, it's an adventure to create something new... It's very enriching for my own life. It's made me a life-long student.

I involve my coworkers in singing, dancing, and improvisation. It has doubled the energy in the circle with the residents by getting staff involved, and it's become part of the culture of both places. It boosts the morale of the whole environment, creates stronger relationships among the staff, and creates stronger relationships between the staff and the residents.

And I still use puppets. After Emilou, one of my favorite residents, passed on, I got permission from her family to have a puppet made that was based on her. Emilou is my sidekick, and she always comes with me. All the residents love Emilou. She blows kisses to every single resident before we start, and she always says, "I didn't know I had so many friends." I always seat her in an empty chair between people. They expect her – they love her. She's probably a real endorphin-releasing agent. She elicits more smiles than I do. She gets a reaction from everyone she blows a kiss to. She's been a real unexpected development in my work… she even has her own Facebook page: Emilou Goldenpuppet. If you want to see some of the work that we do together – Emilou, residents, staff, and I – please visit!

DISCOVERING MUSIC THERAPY

▶ by Teri K. Holmberg

Teri K. Holmberg, MA, MT-BC received a Bachelor of Music degree from the University of North Texas and a Master of Arts (music therapy) degree from Texas Woman's University. She has provided music therapy services to special education classes in Texas, Michigan, and Kansas. She is currently retired.

Starting Out

I began my career in the early 1990s as a general music teacher at a school that served students living in low-income housing. As a result, many of my students were struggling with emotional and developmental issues that often come with a lack of financial stability. Some students were emotionally withdrawn, some had significant behavioral issues, while others were substantially behind their peers academically. I noticed that it was often difficult for these students to focus on my instruction and realized that unless and until these issues were addressed, they would be a continuing barrier to my students' academic success.

As a music educator, I was not trained to help students overcome these barriers. My lack of knowledge was further impeded by an almost total absence of information-sharing between classroom teachers, parents, administrators, and myself. Unlike the classroom teacher, I was not provided with relevant information regarding my students' challenges or special needs and had to insist that I have access to student files. It would be an understatement to say that it was very frustrating to know that I was expected to teach students without being provided with crucial information regarding their specific needs.

Although gaining additional information was helpful in understanding the underlying factors behind some of my students' learning difficulties, I was still not equipped to effectively address them. My training focused on techniques to teach and develop musical skills. I was not a therapist or special education teacher, and I knew that my attempts to help my students with special needs, while earnest, were not adequate.

Discovering Music Therapy

During the struggle to better serve my students, I met a music therapist purely by chance. I had never heard of music therapy, but her description of her work with students in special education opened my eyes to the possibility of using music as a tool to develop other kinds of skills essential to success in life. After teaching music for two years, I decided to return to school and pursue a master's degree in music therapy in the hope of learning how to more effectively assist children with the types of needs I had encountered as a music teacher.

Although this was not typical in the United States at the time, the area in which I lived employed a large number of music therapists to work in the public-school districts, and I was very fortunate to have many opportunities while in school to observe and work with a number of excellent music therapists who specialized in providing music therapy for children and young adults with a variety of developmental disabilities. I decided that this area of specialization was a good fit for me since I had a background in education.

Music Therapy Internship

Upon completion of my coursework, I applied for an internship position at the Denton State School. It had once been a residential school for children with special needs until the mid-1970s, but with the change of policy to include all children in public schools, the current residents were all adults who had lived there since childhood. At the time there were no public-school music therapy internships available in my area, so this was the best fit for my area of specialization.

The residents at the State School ranged from people with severe multiple impairments who were non-verbal and used wheelchairs to people with significant physical impairments, but little to no intellectual disabilities. Some residents were surprisingly musically gifted. Learning how to adapt therapeutically beneficial musical experiences for people with such a wide range of needs and abilities proved to be the biggest challenge of my work there.

For some residents, their biggest need was one-on-one human interaction which did not involve some kind of care-taking. My first experience with the most impaired residents of the school was overwhelming. My co-intern and I were taken by our supervisor into a large room where thirty to forty residents were waiting for their weekly music therapy session. They were all in wheelchairs, none of them could speak, and many had very limited range of movement. They required around-the-clock care for all of their physical needs. The medications they took caused constant drooling, so the smell in the room was horrible, and some seemed totally unresponsive. I remember wondering how I was ever going to be able to do anything that could help them. My supervisor played songs on a keyboard while my co-intern and I sang and went from person to person and tried to engage them in an interaction. For some, this involved playing a simple percussion instrument, such as a maraca or a tambourine. For others, it meant making eye contact while we sang to them. As I moved from person to person, I quickly realized that the musical experience was a means of allowing for an authentic, normal interaction, not between a therapist and a client, but between two human beings. When I sang or played an instrument with each person, their smiles and attentiveness were an acknowledgement of a positive, life-affirming event which spoke to the essential humanity in everyone. It was a profoundly humbling experience, and one which I have never forgotten.

Getting Started in Music Therapy

Music therapy with children in special education

After completion of my internship, I applied for two part-time music therapy positions: one serving special education students at a public school and the other at a children's hospital. It was unusual at the time to have open music therapy positions so readily available; many music therapists still had to create their own jobs by convincing various institutions to hire them. Since I lived in a highly populated metropolitan area that had largely embraced music therapy as a valuable service, it was much easier to find employment. I was hired for both positions as an independent contractor, which meant that I became a small business owner as a sole practitioner. I had to set rates for my services, bill my employers for services rendered, keep books on my business, and file taxes as a business owner. I liked the independence of being my own boss, but it required more financial discipline than as an employee of someone else's business. I had to budget my income to pay quarterly taxes, and I had to save for retirement and insurance, as I received no benefits from my employers.

Although both of my new jobs as a music therapist involved working with children, the needs of my clients were often very different. In the school setting, the focus of music therapy was helping students achieve developmental goals such as focusing attention, developing communication and language skills, and attaining pre-academic skills so that they could be as successful and independent as possible at school and beyond. At the hospital, the focus of therapy was on normalization and control, pain management, and minimization of developmental regression. In other words, my job was to help the kids be kids as much as possible in a very abnormal environment for children.

The most surprising thing I learned from working with the students in my special education classrooms was that often music therapy interventions, instead of "teaching" students new skills, served as a vehicle for removing barriers to students' ability to demonstrate skills they already had. It was a matter of finding an effective way of adapting instruction to their needs and abilities that allowed them to be successful. Music often became the "key" to unlocking what was already inside them. This was most apparent in students with challenges in communicating, as in children with autism. Music frequently served as an effective means of both understanding and expressing information, and once the barrier to communication was removed, it was amazing to discover what these students could actually do. This taught me a valuable lesson. I tried never to assume limitations on my students' abilities or put a ceiling on what they could accomplish.

Music therapy with children in the hospital

As for the music therapy position at the hospital, far more was required of me in adapting music therapy interventions to the frequently shifting requirements of my clients. Some children were only in the hospital for brief stays. Some had chronic conditions which required frequent visits. Some children were terminally ill. The medical condition of a child could change dramatically from day to day. I often did not know who I would be treating or the condition of the children I would be seeing until I came into work.

For the children who were in the hospital briefly, I had to conduct an assessment of their needs, develop a treatment plan, and execute music therapy interventions during the course of a few hours. Objectives had to be very short-term and outcomes immediate. For children with more serious conditions which required an extended hospital stay, I was able to develop a more comprehensive treatment plan, which might include a number of long- and short-term objectives. Regardless of the length of their stay, the patients at the hospital had much more input into the activities and objectives of music therapy sessions than the students I served in public schools. Part of the reason for this was the comprehension and intellectual ability of the patients, and part was the need of these patients to feel a sense of control over part of their lives.

Hospital stays involve many unpleasant experiences over which patients have no control, so it was very important as much as possible to let patients direct the therapy. My primary role was to offer a variety of musical experiences and invite patients to participate in the activities that most appealed to them. This was especially important during painful procedures. I always made a plan with the patient before a painful procedure, but I would change the plan according to the patient's direction as they were receiving treatment. As a result, I learned to be very flexible as a therapist during my time at the children's hospital.

My work at the children's hospital was also more emotionally demanding than in the public schools. I was interacting with children and parents who were often experiencing the most frightening and traumatic events of their lives. The children were withdrawn, and the parents were stressed. The situations I encountered were often very sad. I had to walk a fine line between investing emotionally in the families I worked with and maintaining professional distance so I could be an effective therapist. In order to achieve this balance, I kept my focus completely on the immediate needs of the patients and their families during sessions. After work, I allowed myself to decompress and process the emotions I felt about each patient, and sometimes I had to grieve their loss. These experiences showed me that I could be strong for others when they needed me, but I could get close to my clients without compromising my effectiveness as a therapist. It also taught me the importance of self-care. I had to allow for a time and place to heal from the emotional toll of working in this type of setting.

Starting Over in a New Place

After a few years, my husband accepted a job in a part of the country which was far less populated. In preparation for the move, I researched available music therapy jobs in the area and discovered that not only were there no music therapists working in the entire county, but a music therapist had never worked there. I was facing a much different situation in securing a job than I had when starting my career as a music therapist. I was going to have to create my own job. Since I wanted to continue working in the public-school setting, I made information packets about music therapy in special education and mailed them to every Special Education Director in the county. I called each director and requested meetings. Some refused my requests, while others listened to my presentation about the benefits of music therapy for their students, but told me they didn't have money in their budgets for music therapy services. I made efforts to educate the community by speaking to parent advocacy groups, contacting local media outlets for interviews and conducting free workshops for teachers about music therapy.

After about six months of persistence, I finally convinced one director to hire me. I provided music therapy services to students in twelve different special education classrooms in three different schools. My contract with the school district was as a "consultant to the classroom program," which allowed every student in each classroom to receive music therapy services without a formal assessment and every classroom teacher to receive consultation and training services from me on how to incorporate music interventions into their curriculum. This approach was very well-received by the teachers and other service providers, such as the speech and occupational therapists, who frequently sat in on music therapy sessions in order to observe students' responses and get a clearer picture of students' abilities and needs. This led to a wonderful collaboration between the other therapists and I in which we combined our interventions with students. For example, I wrote songs for the speech therapists which focused on particular sounds or words they were working on in therapy, and they taught me different oral motor exercises that the students needed to work on which I incorporated into music activities in my sessions. Sometimes we combined our therapy sessions and worked with the students together. This integrated approach to therapy allowed for more consistency in therapeutic interventions and provided repeated reinforcement of the skills we were helping the students attain. In other words, they had more opportunities to learn, which led to more efficient instruction from the therapists and better skill retention for the students.

As word of my services in the area spread and parents became interested in getting music therapy for their children, I began to receive a number of requests for formal music therapy assessments from special education directors all over the county. Prior to this time, I had very little experience with conducting assessments in order to determine whether or not a child qualified for district-funded music therapy. There were a few diagnostic models available at that time for assessments, and I could apply the general outline they provided, but I found that every situation was so unique that I had to develop a very specific assessment process customized to each student I evaluated. The musical interventions had to be specifically designed to fit the needs of each student in order for the assessment to yield valid results.

Since I was the only practicing music therapist within three counties, conducting assessments posed an ethical issue; if an assessment determined that a student qualified for services, then I was the only person who could reasonably provide the service. This created a situation with potential for a conflict of interest. I addressed this problem in several ways. First, I notified all administrators about the potential conflict before I agreed to conduct an assessment. Second, I took extremely detailed notes of any interviews or observations I conducted and included them in my reports. Lastly, I either recorded all interactions with each student (if I was given legal permission) or had a witness in the room who could take notes and corroborate the information that I provided in my report. This was not an ideal situation, but I found that lots of details and corroborated data was reassuring to administrators and protected me from ethical concerns.

Universal Truths about Working as a Therapist

Although the experiences at each of the jobs I had in my early years as a music therapist were very different in some ways, they all taught me some universal truths about work as a therapist:

- First, you cannot have the attitude that you are going to "fix" someone. All you can do is present opportunities and serve as a guide for change. If the client doesn't respond the way you hoped, it is up to you to figure out what to adjust so that they are getting what they need to be successful.
- Second, it is absolutely necessary to be flexible during sessions. Planning is essential, but therapists must take direction from the responses and immediate needs of their clients and adjust accordingly.
- Third, the development and maintenance of good musical skills is absolutely imperative. It is very difficult to be an effective music therapist if you are not a well-trained musician with confidence in your musical abilities. Your focus has to be on the client, not the chord progressions you are playing on the guitar. You may often have to improvise, compose, or transpose during a session, and you must have the skills to do so.
- Fourth, you must maintain good emotional health to be an effective therapist. Music therapy is often an emotionally demanding job which requires a high level of emotional intimacy between client and therapist. Self-care and support from other music therapists is very helpful in sustaining the balance between intimacy and professionalism.
- Fifth, make sure that you can be an effective advocate for your profession. You will frequently be asked to explain what you do. Prepare yourself with a good answer, regardless of who asks the question. A stranger or acquaintance might only need a short response that provides a brief summary. A potential employer needs a more detailed answer which gives them a better understanding about the science behind and benefits of music therapy.
- Lastly, remember that all people are musical beings and that, regardless of background or ability, music is a universal phenomenon that everyone can and should experience. Always appreciate the beauty in that truth.

FINDING MY PURPOSE IN LIFE

▶ An Interview With Sarah Edwards

Sarah Edwards, MA, RDT works for Friends Life Community in Nashville, Tennessee. She graduated from Kansas State University in 2017 with her MA in drama therapy.

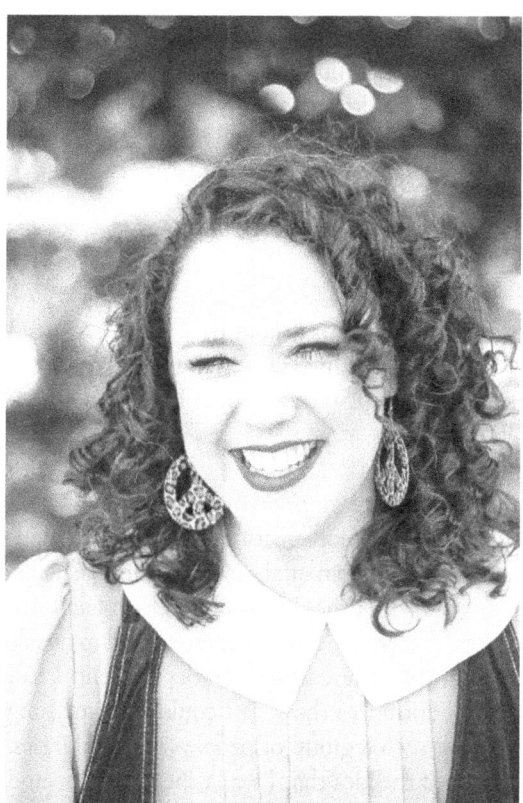

Figure 1.5 Drama Therapist Sarah Edwards.

Which came first – your interest in theatre or your interest in working with people with intellectual and developmental disabilities?

Definitely theatre was first. I'm from a very rural area in Tennessee and didn't start really being a part of the theatre world until I was in seventh grade. The Dixie Carter

Performing Arts Center in Huntington gave me a place to explore the creative space that was within me. Then I considered myself an entertainer, and I dove into acting and dancing and performing of all kinds. Through the arts I found my true self. I was, "OK, I want to do this as a career!" I didn't know what that was going to be, but I knew I wanted to go to college for theatre. I wasn't sure if I wanted to major in performance or education, but then I found Belmont University in Nashville, loved the program, and committed to theatre education because I felt like that would be more stable than the performance route. I'm a very spontaneous person, but I also need stability. I thought I could teach, and I could also entertain on the side.

Working with people with intellectual and developmental disabilities (IDD) started early on, too. I worked with a girl with autism for about 2 ½ years while I was in high school. She was nonverbal. I really enjoyed that. I had never been around anyone with intellectual disabilities before. Actually, her mother was the first person that put into my brain that I could connect working with people with disabilities and theatre. She suggested that to me when I was in tenth grade. It is a challenge when you kind of sort of know what you want to do, but you aren't sure how to do it.

When you were getting ready to graduate from college, what was your plan?

I student-taught the last semester of my senior year and at that point I realized that I did not like the traditional classroom setting. Loved the kids, loved the community, but I didn't like the school setting. So that's when I asked my mentor at the time, what should I do now?

Actually, it just so happened that the first semester of my senior year, I got a work-study position at Friends Life Community with people with disabilities. It's a nonprofit that provides services for adults with developmental disabilities in Nashville. I loved it! I had never worked with anyone with other kinds of developmental disabilities than the girl in high school. At the same time, that semester I had to decide what my senior show was going to be in the theatre education department. I had options: I could direct a show, I could perform in a show, or I could do something different. This was my first time working with a group of people with disabilities. The executive director at Friends Life loved the idea that I was a theatre major, and she loved the idea of my doing something for my senior project with them. I was terrified. In three months, we created a very short, very low-risk performance that was based off of a theatre game called Freeze Dance.

I did that first semester, and I had to say goodbye to go do my student teaching. Then I realized that I didn't want to teach in the school system, and I thought, "What am I going to do?" My mentor and I talked a lot about my options. I came to the conclusion that grad school was my best bet, because I wanted to help people through theatre – that was louder to me and more attractive than being on the stage myself. Even though I was terrified doing that performance at Friends Life, doing it absolutely rocked my world. I had never experienced anything like that, and I knew the possibilities were endless in that realm.

How did you know the possibilities would be endless?

I knew it because these particular people at Friends Life had never been in a show, but their motivation, excitement, and presence within those three months were so bold. They were changed because of the performance. That made it even more loud to me. It changed them, and it changed me, and their families, and the audience members! They had never seen anything like this before. I got a job at Friends Life after I graduated and started teaching life skills through drama for two years.

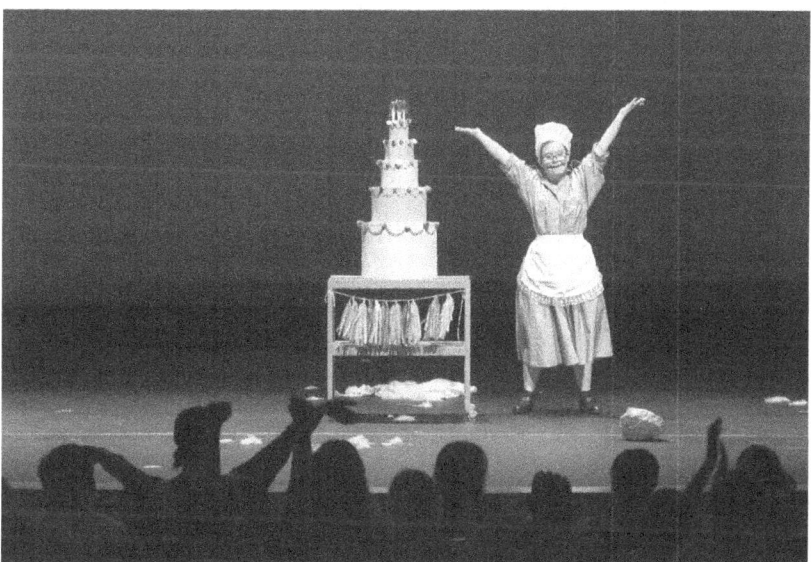

Figure 1.6 Photo from the play *Recipes for Life*, created by Advocacy Through the Arts. Friends Life Community provides teenagers and adults with intellectual and developmental disabilities opportunities to grow personally, develop socially, and be active members of the greater community. One of FLC's programs, Advocacy Through the Arts, serves to empower individuals with disabilities to tell their own unique stories. This program allows each Friend to discover their voice, tell their story, and connect with others through a shared experience.

What made you decide to go to graduate school?

I realized I needed more skills. I had kept in touch with my mentor, and she said, "You've got two options: drama therapy or applied theatre." First, I toured USC (University of Southern California) for their applied theatre program in 2014. There were several things that stood out to me: What I liked was that at the end they would take all their students to a village in South America and use theatre to support the village in skills – and that was really cool. But it was only a one-year program, and I wondered if that would be long enough to teach me what I needed to know. Plus, it was $60,000 a year. There were no graduate assistantships and nothing to support you as a student, and it's expensive to live in Los Angeles.

Then I came to visit the drama therapy program at K-State. You were warm, but you weren't pushy. You just gave me information and let me make up my mind. I knew from your email and conversation with you that I was going to get a lot of opportunity to work with people with disabilities, but I would get experience with other people, too, so I would get skills to work with other populations. And K-State had graduate assistantships. After coming to visit, I was sold.

I got a graduate assistantship working at the Hoeflin Stone House which was the experimental childcare center on campus run by the early childhood program. Working at a preschool was the hardest job of my life! Nap time was the hardest thing: trying to get 3- or 4-year-olds to take a nap! What I loved about that job, though, was I was able to do drama therapy with the children every day. Every day was an opportunity to use what I was learning in class.

What difference has your degree made to the work that you do now?

First, the quality of my work has increased tremendously. I started off at Friends Life in my senior year with very low-risk theatre work because I didn't feel that I really knew what I was doing. When I graduated, I went back to work for Friends Life because they really wanted me. After graduate school, I have had the bravery to push my actors and to challenge myself, because I have skills. Because of my degree, I learned how my own creative process works in situations that are one-on-one, that are with groups, and that work with creating performances.

What I've been doing has been successful for my clients, for me personally, and for the vision of the organization that I work with. Because of my degree I've had the confidence to start a dance ensemble, a traveling acting troupe, and a collaboration with the visual arts specialist to do a year-long performance piece integrating all the arts. Without the degree there is no way, no way I would be able to do as much as I've done so far. Finding my process has given me bravery.

The reason why I get to keep building and creating programming goes back to the things I learned in school. Everything I've been doing is making an impact for the board members, clients, families, and audiences. The executive director at Friends Life keeps wanting drama therapy opportunities to expand.

I think my work has given me impact on the community in Nashville. I also started an access program at the Dixie Carter Performing Arts Center to include people with disabilities in their programs. They are learning about people with disabilities in a bigger way. Neurotypical audiences who see our traveling troupe from Friends Life are entertained, and it's high-quality entertainment so they want us to come to perform at luncheons and conferences.

Now I understand the need for ethics in the service work and the drama therapy work I do. Before I went to K-State, the concept of ethics didn't exist for me. No one talked about it. Not at undergraduate school, not in teaching, not on the job at Friends Life or at Dixie Carter. I'm now teaching my teaching artists, Friends Life staff, and volunteers about making sure the clients are protected and treated with dignity, safety, and confidentiality.

I have discovered that a lot of my clients have had traumatic experiences with sexual abuse. I am making sure I have a support system put in place for those

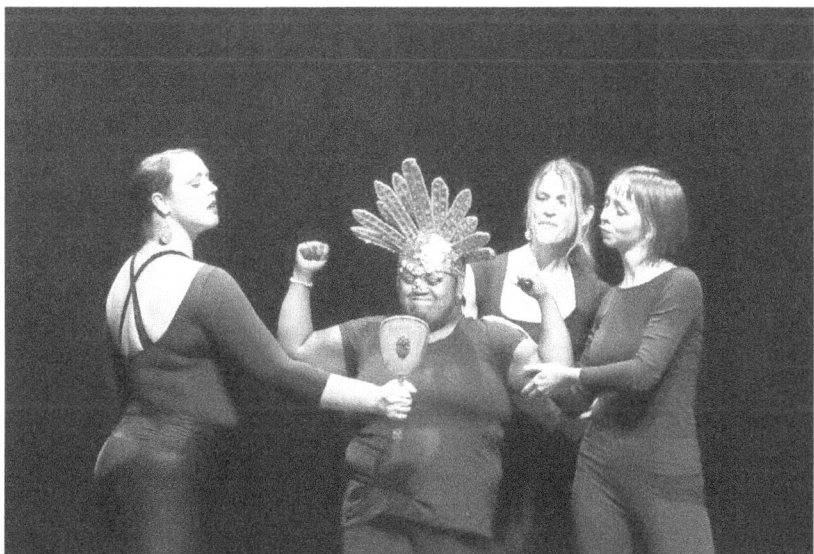

Figure 1.7 Photo from the play *I Love You*, created by Advocacy Through the Arts, a Friends Life Community production.

people. I have had to educate the staff about how important trauma-informed care is and how to do it. They had no idea how often people with disabilities are abused, and they were in the disability field.

The other thing that came out of my degree in drama therapy is my responsibility to advocate for the integrity of people with disabilities. It goes back to the quality of the shows we create; I use integrity, sophistication, and dignity when we are creating a performance. We are really trying to break down the stigma that adults with IDD face – that they are less than people who are neurotypical. We also need to teach that they are not children. They are colorful, unique, quirky, and playful individuals in ways that many people who are neurotypical aren't anymore. My job is to meet in the middle. To let the actors present themselves as colorful and playful, to allow their magical spirits to come alive, but to never let them appear childish.

At Friends Life we treat them like adults and make sure their experience is adult. As actors I hold them to the highest standards. I tell them in rehearsals, "You are going to learn these lines, and you are going to project loudly enough that everyone in the audience can hear you." They do in-depth character work. The integrity goes to setting high expectations. And pushing them. That is true equality.

MOVEMENT INITIATION: BEGINNING A CAREER IN DANCE/ MOVEMENT THERAPY

▶ by Mariah Meyer LeFeber

Mariah Meyer LeFeber, MA, LPC, BC-DMT is a Portland, Oregon-based dance/movement therapist and counselor. She infuses her passion for DMT into her work as a counselor, educator, and supervisor. Her best teachers (and dance partners) are her husband and two daughters.

Intersectionality

In 1989, professor Kimberlé Crenshaw coined the term *intersectionality*. The term describes how gender, race, class, and other identities and/or characteristics "intersect" with one another, overlapping and mutually impacting each other (Crenshaw, 1989). Born out of Crenshaw's work in ideas related to critical race theory, intersectionality was officially added to the Oxford Dictionary in 2015 and gained widespread attention a few years later during the January 2017 Women's March. At its core, the term suggests that individual identities intersect, and this intersection impacts how people are treated, understood, and viewed (Crenshaw, 1989). The term illustrates how each of our individual stories arise out of a beautiful myriad of intersecting parts. The following pages are the story of my ever-evolving awareness of my own intersectional identity and how, along this path of exploration, I found my way to the field of dance/movement therapy (DMT). My hope is that my story will inspire you to think about your own identities, about the lessons you've already learned, and the truths you are building towards, even now as you read.

Starting Out

I was born in the Pacific Northwest, the daughter of a pastor and a music teacher. Before I turned one, my family moved to the heart of the Midwest

– back to where my parents had both been raised on farms in Nebraska. My three siblings and I grew up on these rolling plains, and certainly the seeds for my story were planted there. I grew up dancing, taking classes at a local dance studio where I would spend much of my time come high school, as a member of my high school dance team, and in the basement of my house, choreographing lament-filled solos to the *Legends of the Fall* soundtrack. I didn't know then how this growing love for movement would fuel me going forward.

I left home to attend college at the University of Minnesota – Twin Cities. There, I declared a double major: one in dance – not because I truly thought I'd have a career in the field but because I felt I just couldn't quit doing what I loved – and a second in psychology, which I had become very interested in thanks to some excellent classes and teachers in high school. One clear truth that emerged then and has continued to develop was my love for (and fascination with the science of) people; engaging in the study of people has allowed me to more fully embrace, engage with, and love humanity.

Only a few months into my first semester of college, I found myself terribly overwhelmed, questioning how to possibly balance the expectations of two programs. I sought advice from my general advisor. It was she who asked me if I had ever heard of dance/movement therapy. She then suggested that the field might be one where I could find a way to integrate my passions (and identities) as opposed to seeing them as competing entities. I went back to my dorm room and pulled out the piece of paper where my advisor had scrawled down the website for the national organization and spent hours that night poring over the information (which, admittedly, took longer than it would today, due to the speed of internet in the early 2000s). Clichés aside, it is true that the body doesn't lie, and in that moment, I felt deep in my gut this was the work I wanted to do with my life.

I would spend the rest of my undergraduate career fitting my circular desire to pursue dance/movement therapy into the two square pegs of my areas of study. This wasn't easy at times – often making sacrifices in one content area for the sake of the other – yet as I became more aware of and settled into my intersecting identities, my path forward became increasingly clear. What I learned in my early searching is a truth that lingers still today: there are mentors in this field who will encourage and support you to write your own story. Several incredible dance professors – while not Dance Movement Therapists (dmts) – modeled for me how to meet your client (student) where they are and help them to grow and build from their strengths, a fundamentally connecting approach that I would later learn was also a key tenet in DMT. My dance advisor supported me through the application and research process of pursuing an undergraduate research grant to further study DMT and encouraged me to take the one introduction to DMT elective offered in the department. Finally, the local chapter of dance therapists welcomed me whole-heartedly. I attended some of their chapter meetings, and one in particular met with me and allowed me to shadow her work doing dance therapy on a psychiatric inpatient unit. This mentorship, encouragement, and practical engagement all made me believe that my dream was tangible, and thus these are gifts that I try to embody and pass on today to others who also find themselves in this place of exploration and anticipation.

Sticking It Out: Graduate School

I applied to a handful of the approved DMT graduate programs during my final year of undergraduate studies. After my acceptance to Columbia College Chicago, I ended up moving back home to Nebraska and deferring my admittance. During that gap year, I worked various jobs that built my resume in unexpected ways, fell in love, and lived at home trying to help as my father succumbed to a cancer-ridden body. I include this part of my story because it is just as true and important as the others – who I have become as a dance/movement therapist cannot be separated from who I am as a person – as I believe is true for all of us who pursue this healing and heartfelt work.

Following my year in Nebraska, I moved to Chicago and started the dual master's degree program in dance/movement therapy and counseling at Columbia College Chicago. My two and half years in the intensive program shaped me in ways that could never be captured in words. In the world of therapy, we often talk about the implicit healing power of the therapeutic relationship – and it was the relationships I made while studying that taught and healed me simultaneously. Not only did I learn from wise professor/researcher/clinicians, but I also learned daily from my cohort of peers. In this place I gained the roots needed to be able to grow and eventually spread my professional wings.

As is the case across the board in healing professions, my clinical internship experiences – first for an inpatient child and adolescent psychiatric unit in Chicago and then for the Hancock Center for Dance/Movement Therapy in Madison, WI – provided educational experiences for me that never could have been matched inside of classroom walls. It was in these settings that the practice of working with real clients (versus role-playing with classmates in courses) came to life and where I truly grasped the simultaneous beauty and brokenness of moving with someone through their pain.

Finding Success

Upon the completion of my degree, living full-time in Madison, WI, I started looking in earnest for my first job as a freshly minted dance/movement therapist. Throughout my studies, I learned that an essential skill for flourishing as a creative arts therapist was learning how to talk about the work in a way that others could relate to and understand. There is a language within the field of DMT, and that language must be thoughtfully translated to help others outside of the niche understand the potential and power of the work. I believe it was my ability to translate in this way, along with my passion, aided by the beautiful luck of being interviewed by an art therapist, that landed me a full-time job working at a clinic for children with autism and other developmental delays.

My work at this clinic, nearly fifteen years ago now as I sit and write this essay, introduced me to a community of incredible, comprehensively trained, and uniquely skilled mental health professionals. I added them to my growing network of fellow dmts and mentors, and those relationships have continued to develop and support me through rich and varied vocational experiences. In addition to clinical work with children, adults, and families, I've been fortunate to expand my work into the training and supervision of emerging counselors and dance/movement therapists. In its own circuitous dance, my path has led me out of the Midwest and back to the Pacific Northwest, where I continue to engage and explore my contributions to the field. While I could tell you about the gifts and quirks of each of my vocational experiences, perhaps it is most fitting to speak to a few guiding ideas that have led the way for me in my journey.

The Importance of Process Over Product

When I was in graduate school, one mantra that we were reminded of frequently was the concept of *process over product*. Like many of us in DMT and the creative arts therapies in general, I came to the work from a performance-based background. It took years for me to fully grasp that the beauty and power of DMT work has very little to do with a movement product and very much to do with the process and the movement that brought you through. Holding on to the principle of process over product has guided me in my vocation, and more importantly, has offered me a lens for living. The fields of DMT and counseling have shifted and changed exponentially since my own educational experience, and a growth mindset, focused on process, has supported me to continue growing and changing as well. For me, believing in this work is believing that I will never have arrived – but that I'll always be swimming in the midst of the magnificent and messy process.

Irmgard Bartenieff, a physical therapist known for her contributions to the field of DMT, presented a concept she referred to often and called the *movement lemniscate*, or the lively interplay that "*inner connectivity breeds outer expressivity*" (Hackney, 2002, p. 34). In DMT theory, we understand this to mean that the more integration we experience on an internal level, the more expressivity we have access to in our bodies and words on an external level. Essentially, our inner connectivity exists in an ever-evolving, co-creating relationship with our outer expressivity. I've watched my own clients grow from making these internal connections to building their own personal sense of self and, finally, to extending their identities out into their relationships and their work in the world. This flowing, embodied integration allows us to be in a feedback loop with ourselves, where we can check in with our own internal experience. That reflection, in turn, influences the external world, which, in return, reflects and influences us back. A driving force for me as I encounter each unique client, student, or supervisee, is to walk alongside them as they build their own personal identity kaleidoscope, a lemniscate of inner and outer connectivity.

According to psychiatrist Daniel Siegel, neural integration occurs when the experiences between the brain, mind, and relationship are linked coherently. One might say that Siegel's concept of neural integration allows space for the developing process and also speaks to the lemniscate of internal and external connectivity. Neuroscience suggests that the linkage of specialized and differentiated parts leads to a brain that integrates top to bottom/left to right, flows with flexibility, and results in neuroplasticity – or the brain's ability to grow, adapt, and change (Siegel, 2012). The language of neuroscience captures for me how in my own work and life, much like the integrated mind, I find myself in the process of *linking my differentiated parts*. To pursue a career as a dmt is to constantly be considering and integrating your intersectional identities and your differentiated parts. As I understand my own unique identity as a dance/movement therapist, I can further integrate and work connected to helpers and healers everywhere.

Conclusion

One final lesson I will leave you with is this: *movement initiates from somewhere.* When I was a college dance major, I had a professor who led us in an initiation warm-up exercise. We would move across the dance studio with different parts of our bodies leading and initiating, or starting, the movement – initiating and then propelling motion from one side of the room to the other through the crown of our head, elbows, scapula, pelvis, and so on. In the moment, that improvisational exercise reminded me that movement initiation comes in many forms and from many different sources. While I might be stuck in my own habitual, every day, embodied patterns, movement begins from somewhere deep within, initiates, and then moves out into countless different ripples and designs. My own story of initiation led me to the path of dance/movement therapy, and I'm so glad to have found a home in this work. Wherever you find yourself today, I encourage you to slow down, take a long, deep breath, and notice where your own movement is initiating from – and then allow that movement to nudge you forward. Trust that your body will lead the way.

References

Hackney, P. (2002). *Making connections: Total body integration through Bartenieff Fundamentals*. Routledge.

Crenshaw, K. (1989). Demarginalizing the intersection of race and sex: A black feminist critique of antidiscrimination doctrine, feminist theory and antiracist politics. *University of Chicago Legal Forum, 1989*(1), Article 8.

Siegel, D. (2012). *The developing mind: How relationships and the brain interact to shape who we are*. Guilford Publications, Inc.

MULTICULTURAL REPRESENTATIONS IN THE CREATIVE ARTS THERAPIES: ART THERAPISTS OF COLOR MATTER

▶ by Denise Boston

Denise Boston, RDT, PhD (she/her/hers) has over twenty-five years of experience as an educational and health equity consultant, culturally responsive organizational coach, educator, and community-based research specialist. She previously served as Dean of Diversity and Inclusion and core faculty at the California Institute of Integral Studies. Her most recent work is with the Key of Life: Re-animating Teaching and Learning as senior associate. Denise earned her BFA in drama from the University of North Carolina School of the Arts, her MA in psychology and counseling from Goddard College, and her PhD in counseling psychology from Walden University.

> *When every culture is honored and valued, more*
> *accessibility and communal wellness are generated.*
> — Kiona Medina, Expressive Arts Therapist/
> Practitioner

The purpose of this chapter is to shed light as to why representation in the Creative Arts Therapy field matters. My intention is to 1) expound on the clinical practices, scientific evidence, and notions about Creative Arts Therapies; 2) highlight the historical context of creative arts healing practices in Black, Brown, and Indigenous value systems; and 3) encourage aspiring counselors and community-based arts activists of color to consider bringing their passion and talents to the Creative Arts Therapy field.

A Career in Creative Activism

My career has continuously taken me back and forth between creative community activism and higher education. These aims never seemed at odds with one another. Creative activism, for me, entails aesthetically addressing racial, health, and educational inequalities, while academia offers intellectual rigor, peer-to-peer learning, and a community of inquiry. I find them complimentary in my quest to use the arts in the healing and research process as well as confronting injustice in all its forms. In my dual roles as an expressive arts therapy scholar and community informed practitioner, I have witnessed how social and emotional learning occurs through arts-based encounters as well as measurable shifts in critical consciousness and self-actualization. I have discovered in my work as an arts practitioner in schools, homeless shelters, senior centers, and prisons – primarily with people of African descent – how powerful the arts are in providing a healing space to explore and re-envision a multitude of human explorations, social connections, and transformative growth experiences.

From a social justice and racial equity lens, my career path has led to increased efforts to address social determinants of mental health and uncover the root cause of disease and toxic stress in underserved communities through radical creative interventions – ensuring that all Black, Indigenous, People of Color and other marginalized groups have a fair and just opportunity to live healthy, purposeful, and optimal lives. Ultimately, I could not have anticipated how significant my representation as a Black author, teacher, social activist, and art-based researcher would be in academia, and, more particularly, in the creative arts therapies field. This essay explores why representation in the creative arts therapy profession matters and the ways in which a culturally relevant environment enhances the healing process in communities of color.

The Creative Arts Therapies Field

Psychology is one mental health field that has many specialties (e.g., counseling psychology, school psychology, forensic psychology, developmental psychology), and continues to evolve with new branches that are emerging to keep up with current domestic and global issues and recognition of persistent disparities in mental health (McGuire & Miranda, 2008). In many branches of psychology, there has been a growing interest in the process of art-making and expressive therapies to enhance the therapeutic encounter and the mental health and well-being of children, youth, and adults (McNiff, 2004).

According to Malchiodi (2005), expressive therapies are defined as the use of art, music, dance/movement, drama, poetry/creative writing, play, and media, with the context of psychotherapy, counseling, rehabilitation, or health care. Research trends support the application of the creative arts within diverse settings. An aesthetic therapeutic presence has the opportunity to improve the delivery of healthcare and facilitate an experience wherein imagination, cognition, and affect are effectively engaged (Sajnani et al., 2020). Aesthetic approaches value the place of the creativity in human life. According to Levine (2005), this aesthetic mindset draws on the power of the imagination in areas such as role plays, active imagination, and free association. Various art disciplines offer an integrated blend of classroom, experiential learning, and creative therapy specialties.

The creative arts therapy professional journey traditionally begins at an approved licensure track graduate level and provides a synthesis of creative, aesthetic, and psychotherapeutic theory and practice. Master level counseling programs in universities across the country may have arts-based therapeutic concentrations in areas of Dance/Movement Therapy, Drama Therapy, Music Therapy, Poetry Therapy, Expressive Arts Therapy, and Art Therapy. Arts-based counseling courses offer an in-depth theoretical framework that integrates philosophical and experiential learning forms; aesthetic decision-making in clinical work and creative processes, such as drawing, creative movement, and drama, to explore the ways in which individuals of all ages, ethnic backgrounds, and cultural orientations express thoughts and feelings in a manner that is different than only by verbal means (Malchiodi, 2005).

Upon completion of coursework and a clinical practicum placement, graduates are eligible to pursue state licensure or non-clinical arts-based services areas, such as education, personal growth, social justice, and cooperative settings. Creative arts therapists and practitioners also have an opportunity to join the various creative arts associations, such as the North American Drama Therapy Association (NADTA), American Music Therapy Association (AMTA), and International Expressive Arts Therapy Association (IEATA).

Creative Arts Therapy: Why Representation Matters

Therapy that recognizes institutional racism and cultural wounding as trauma helps to address mental health disparities in communities of color (Williams et al., 2018; Woods-Jaeger et al., 2018). According to Williams (2019), racial trauma is due to the debilitating effect of racism and discrimination that Black, Brown, and Indigenous people experience after being exposed either directly or indirectly. The US Department of Health and Human Services (USDHHS, 2001) asserts that people of color are less likely to seek treatment for mental health issues than whites, are more likely to end treatment early, and would prefer seeing a therapist who is of similar race or ethnicity as his/her/their selves. As ethnocultural diversity in the United States grows and vulnerable communities face equitable health care and health disparities, efforts are needed to better understand social determinants and circumstances by which mental health illnesses exist. It is equally important to understand that such determinants define lived experiences by which people are born, educated, live, and work (Marmot & Wilkinson, 2008; Solar & Irwin, 2007).

Among this sociocultural awareness, a top priority must be increased diversity among therapists, which institutes increased representation within the creative arts therapy practice. Unlike verbal psychotherapists, creative arts therapists provide an aesthetic environment embedded in an imaginal context from which to explore and examine emotions as they arise between the client as artist, artmaking, and a reflective witness to what unfolds (Sajnani et al., 2020).

Access to culturally responsive mental health care and culturally relevant diagnostic assessment has been an issue for Black, Brown and Indigenous populations. However, research studies indicate that creative arts therapeutic interventions have been effective in providing restoration and psychological support for children, youth, and adults experiencing depression, loss, anxiety, or posttraumatic stress disorder (PTSD). Art modalities, such as poetry, dance/movement, and storytelling, have contributed toward reducing race-based stress and collective grief, as well as serving as a vehicle toward developing a capacity for radical resilience, healing, and self-empowerment (Boston, 2014; Ganim, 1999; Stuckey & Nobel, 2020).

In this tumultuous time that we are collectively experiencing in the United States, the convergence of the COVID-19 pandemic, structural racism, and policing in communities of color have increased stress and strong emotions in children and adults. The pandemic has rendered visible the disproportionate deaths in the Black, Latinx, and Indigenous communities. According to cultural-centered researchers, a racially motivated stressor overwhelms a person's capacity to cope and a racially motivated, interpersonal severe stressor causes bodily harm or threatens one's life integrity (Bryant-Davis & Ocampo, 2005; Carter, 2007; Loo et al., 2001). The cultural context and psychological toll of pandemic-related racial factors attest to the supposition that representation within the creative arts therapy field matters. By building pathways and intentional pipelines of creative arts therapy practitioners of color, there is potential for utilizing this crisis in closing the gaps and access to mental health engagement, appropriate intervention strategies, and culturally responsive care.

To further offer insight as to why representation of therapists of color in the field of Creative Arts Therapy matters, I reached out to former expressive arts therapy graduate students from the California Institute of Integral Studies. I was honored by their willingness to provide stories and insights of their professional experiences as arts-based licensed marriage and family therapists (MFTs) and practitioners of color. Kiona Medina, Yi-Chen Hsu (a.k.a. Clark), and Tayyibah Chase, represent Columbian, Taiwanese, and African American racial/ethnic identities. Their work as therapists and consultants, both nationally and internationally, is transforming lives by advancing health, wellness, and equality. In relation to the importance of racial/ethnic representation in the Creative Arts Therapy field, I asked them to respond to the following questions:

1) Why does multicultural representation in creative arts therapy careers matter?
2) What difference does it make?
3) What qualities and philosophical underpinnings do you bring to the field?

What they all agreed upon was the healing power of the arts and a need for more mental health providers of color. The following themes were illuminated in their responses:

• Representational presence and the healing process
• Culturally adaptive arts-in-therapy
• Authenticity and trust

Representational presence and the healing process

Partnering with diverse populations entails building a foundation for meaningful and sustainable work. A healing presence is one that includes interpersonal, intrapersonal, and transpersonal connection that leads to therapeutic and/or spiritual exchange within another individual (healee) and also within the healer (McDonough-Means et al., 2004). A wonderful example of an interpersonal community-centered practitioner is Kiona Medina, a Colombian-born expressive arts practitioner/consultant working with children and families in the Bay Area. Kiona states,

While multicultural representation is essential for our communities, if the pathway is not feasible, then it remains an empty ideal. It is in this junction of communal need and social inequality that we have to create what we don't have. Multicultural representation cannot come from the current educational model. We have to reinvent a system where community resources and leadership within our culture create education and a workforce specific to our times and needs. I bring into the field this visionary and resourceful community-centered approach to much-needed social reform. (Personal Communication)

Culturally adaptive arts-in-therapy

Art-making is an integral part of global healing ceremonies and has been used for thousands of years by indigenous cultures throughout the world to create and maintain physical, mental, and spiritual health. Research demonstrates that Africans in the diaspora have a legacy in healing rituals and ceremonies, spirituality, sound/music, dance, storytelling, and visual arts as well as the psychological fortitude needed to sustain and develop self, family, and community in the process of art-making and treating symptoms of psychological distress (DeLoach & Marissa, 2010; Monteiro & Wall, 2011).

Creative arts therapists have the unique opportunity to offer art-based culturally adaptive interventions aligned with the cultural context of their clients or patients. The term "culturally adaptive treatment/interventions" (CAT/I) refers to any modification to evidence-based mental health treatments that involve changes in the approach to service delivery, in the engagement of the therapeutic relationship, or in the components of the intervention itself to accommodate the cultural beliefs, attitudes, and behaviors of the target population (Vinesett et al., 2015; Whaley & Davis, 2007). For example, the Congolese Ngoma ceremony, a healing tradition that uses strong rhythms (drumming) and dance for stress reduction was adapted in a clinical study with US adults with anxiety, depression, and chronic fatigue. Also, the use of drumming has been used as a medium and intervention to address chronic stress and promote social and emotional well-being with youth living in underserved communities (Ho et al., 2011). Clark Hsu, an expressive arts therapist who integrates Eastern spiritual traditions in his healing work asserts:

Creative arts are the unique sound of each soul. When souls meet, harmony occurs, and healing happens. In the meeting of culture or difference, internally or externally, greater potentials are realized. Each culture has a whole heritage and rich array of expressions and artistic instruments. (Personal communication)

Authenticity and trust

The aesthetics of healing, creative agency, and performative literacies are areas of specific culturally informed interventions in marginalised communities available for theoretical and empirical investigation. Irobi (2007) asserts that translocated indigenous African kinesthetic intelligence informs the aesthetics of the indigenous and diasporic perspective. Working with diverse populations requires cultural awareness, historical healing traditions, and strength-based sensibility. Tayyibah Chase is an associate marriage and family therapist in San Francisco, whose mission as a creative arts therapist is to validate the experiences of her clients. She contends,

> There is a level of resonance that is needed for people to trust the therapeutic process and the creative arts help to build that rapport. The use of creative arts for healing is a deeply cathartic process and is more accessible when the client is able to connect with the cultural medium of the art-making processes. There is notable difference when you can connect with the client or community via music, dance, and art that reflects their history and experience. (Personal communication)

Conclusion

Research shows the salient benefits of a diverse creative therapeutic community as well as a culturally adaptive process of art-making to address historical and contemporary racial trauma and social adversities. Even though depression, anxiety, and post-traumatic stress disorder (PTSD) are universal experiences, the ways in which people understand and respond to them are shaped by the attitudes and beliefs of their particular culture and social determinants. Moreover, I hope the voices and personal experiences of current creative therapists and practitioners of color encourage more scholars in this field to conduct theoretically and methodologically congruent research in the area of culturally responsive academic curriculums and equitable educational practicum/internship access. There is a wealth of untapped talent and innovative healing approaches in our communities.

My life has been deeply impacted by a creative arts therapy career and the amazing clients and students I have met along the way. What I know for sure is that art addresses the part of our being that cherishes love, fearlessness, and self-worth. So many opportunities came my way as a performing artist, arts educator, director, arts-based researcher, counselor, administrator, and author because I understood the transformative power of the arts. The expressive arts are universal, and the Creative Arts Therapy field provides an opportunity for aspiring counselors of diverse racial and ethnic backgrounds to infuse experiences of ancestry and the immediate world of their neighborhoods, villages, and indigenous lands into a therapeutic healing space.

References

Boston, D. (2014). *Expressive arts therapy: Responding to traumatic and emotional experiences.* Seven Pillars House of Wisdom. Retrieved from http://www.sevenpillarshouse.org/article/expressive_arts_therapy_responding_to_traumatic_and_emotional_experience

Bryant-Davis, T., & Ocampo, C. (2005). The trauma of racism: Implications for counseling, research, and education. *The Counseling Psychologist, 33*(4), 574–578. doi:10.1177/0011000005276581

Carter, R. T. (2007). Racism and psychological and emotional injury: Recognizing and assessing race-based traumatic stress. *The Counseling Psychologist, 35*(1), 13–105. doi:10.1177/0011000006292033

DeLoach, C., & Marissa, P. (2010). African spiritual methods of healing: The use of Candomblé in traumatic response. *The Journal of Pan African Studies, 3*(8), 40–65.

Ganim, B. (1999). *Art and healing: Using expressive art to heal your body, mind, and spirit.* New World Library.

Ho, P., Tsao, J., Bloch, L., & Zeltzer, L. (2011). The impact of group drumming on social-emotional behavior in low-income children. *Evidence-Based Complementary and Alternative Medicine,* 1–4. doi:10.1093/ecam/neq072

Irobi, E. (2007). What they came with carnival and the persistence of African performance aesthetics in the diaspora. *The Journal of Black Studies, 37*(6), 869–913. doi:10.1177/0021934705283774

Levine, S. (2005). The philosophy of expressive arts therapy: Poiesis as a response to the world. In P. J. Knill, E. G. Levine, & S. Levine (Eds.). *Principles and practice of expressive arts therapy: Toward a therapeutic aesthetic.* (pp. 15–73). Jessica Kingsley Publishers.

Loo, C. M., Fairbank, J. A., Scurfield, R. M., Ruch, L. O., King, D. W., Adams, L. I., & Chentob, D. M. (2001). Measuring exposure to racism: Development and validation of a Race-Related Stress Scale (RRSS) for Asian American Vietnam veterans. *Psychological Assessment, 13*(4), 503–520. doi:10.1037/1040-3590.13.4.503

Malchiodi, C. (2005). Expressive therapies. In C. Malchiodi (Ed.). *Art therapy* (pp. 16–45). Guilford Press.

Marmot, M., & Wilkinson, R. (2008). *Social determinants of health.* Oxford University Press.

McDonough-Means, S., Kreitzer, M., & Bell, I. (2004). Fostering a healing presence and investigating its mediators. *Journal of Alternative and Complementary Medicine, 10*(Supplement 1), S25–S41.

McGuire, T., & Miranda, J. (2008). Racial and ethnic disparities in mental health care: Evidence and policy implications. *Health Affairs, 27*(2), 393–403. doi: 10.1377/hlthaff.27.2.393

McNiff, S. (2004). *Art heals: How creativity cures the soul.* Shambala.

Monteiro, N., & Wall, D. (2011). African dance as healing modality throughout the diaspora: The use of ritual and movement to work through trauma. *The Journal of Pan African Studies, 4*(6), 234–252.

Sajnani, N., Mayor, C., & Tilberg-Webb, H. (2020, July). The role of the arts in education of creative arts therapists in the classroom and online. *The Arts in Psychotherapy, 69*, 101668.

Solar, O., & Irwin, A. (2007). *A conceptual framework for action on the social determinants of health. Discussion paper for the commission on social determinants of health.* Working paper. World Health Organization.

Stuckey, H., & Nobel, J. (2020). The connection between art, healing, and public health: A review of current literature. *American Journal of Public Health, 100*(2), 254–63. doi:10.2105/AJPH.2008.156497

U.S. Department of Health and Human Resources. *Mental health: Culture, race, and ethnicity: A supplement to mental health: A report of the surgeon general.* Retrieved from https://pubmed.ncbi.nlm.nih.gov/20669516/2001

Vinesett, A., Price, M., & Wilson, K. (2015). Therapeutic potential of a drum and dance ceremony based on the African Ngoma tradition. *The Journal of Alternative and Complementary Medicine, 21*(8), 460–465.

Whaley, A., & Davis, K. (2007). Cultural competence and evidenced-based practice in mental health services. *American Psychologist, 62*(6), 563–574. doi:10.1037/0003-066X.62.6.563

Williams, M. T. (2019, February 13). Uncovering the Trauma of Racism. *APA Journals Article Spotlight.* American Psychological Association.

Williams, M., Ching, T., Printz, D., & Wetterneck, C. (2018). Assessing PTSD in ethnic and racial minorities: Trauma and racial trauma. *Directions in Psychiatry, 38*, 179–196.

Woods-Jaeger, B., Cho, B., Sexton, C., Slagel, L., & Goggin, K. (2018). Promoting resilience: Breaking the intergenerational cycle of adverse childhood experiences. *Health Education and Behavior, 45*(5), 772–780. doi:10.1177/1090198117752785

CHAPTER 2

STICKING IT OUT

Sally Bailey, Susan D. Imus, Jason Butler,
Ken neth Aigen, Gaelynn Wolf Bordonaro,
Kathleen Adams, and Danielle Drake

Introduction

Most therapists in the United States have a minimum of a master's degree in order to practice; this is certainly true of creative arts therapists. In undergraduate school, students are usually required to take a wide variety of classes, some in disciplines that they may not have an interest in studying. However, in graduate school, classes solely focus on aspects of the discipline being studied. The essays in this chapter are all written by professors who teach in creative arts therapy master's programs, providing an idea of what courses and types of internships are involved in the different fields of creative arts therapy.

While there are MA programs in Art Therapy, Dance/Movement Therapy, Drama Therapy, Music Therapy, and Expressive Arts Therapies, there are none for Poetry Therapy (also known as Bibliotherapy). Each of the national organizations – The American Art Therapy Association (AATA), The American Dance Therapy Association (ADTA), the North American Drama Therapy Association (NADTA), the American Music Therapy Association (AMTA), the International Expressive Arts Therapy Association (IEATA), and the National Association of Poetry Therapy (NAPT) – set the educational standards for their fields. The schools are required to meet those standards in order to be approved. In the case of NAPT, an alternative training system is set up to train poetry therapists. Kathleen Adams, who runs the Center for Journal Therapy

DOI: 10.4324/9781003035664-2

in Denver, Colorado, is a poetry and journal therapy trainer. She conveys what someone interested in using the written word in therapy would study under the auspices of a trained poetry therapist in order to become a poetry or journal therapist.

The types of courses that students take in creative arts therapy master's degrees have similar categories and structure. Each requires courses in how to use the art (or arts in the case of expressive arts therapies) as therapy, courses in psychology and psychotherapy, at least one course in ethics, and at least one course in research. Ethics are rules set by a professional community to guide decisions related to the care of clients, interactions with colleagues, and the therapist's professional behavior. A course in ethics is crucial for therapists in order to understand how to create appropriate boundaries, stay inside their scope of practice, and do no harm to clients. Research has become more and more important to the creative arts therapy fields in order to prove the efficacy of the work.

All students are required to complete a specific number of internship hours to begin taking the theories they are learning in the classroom and putting them into practice with real human beings. This is never done alone. Early internships – sometimes called practicums – begin with the student working with a credentialed professional in their field. Later, they take on the responsibility of working with groups, families, couples, and/or individuals on their own, with oversight from therapists in the facility in which they are working and weekly supervision with professors at their university.

DRAMA THERAPY EDUCATION

▶ by Jason D. Butler

Jason D. Butler, PhD, RDT-BCT, LCAT is an associate professor and coordinator of the Drama Therapy program at Lesley University. He is a past president of the NADTA and was previously on faculty at Concordia University and New York University. He currently serves as the editor-in-chief of *The Arts in Psychotherapy* (Figure 2.1).

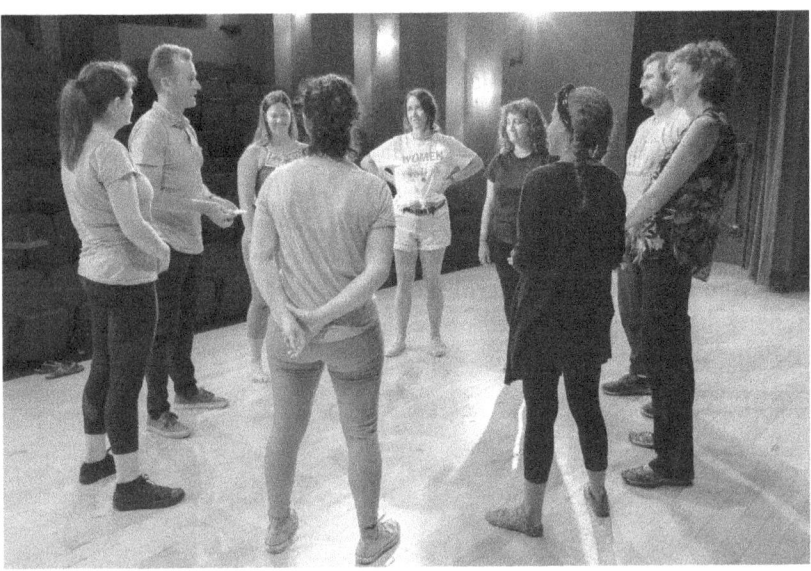

Figure 2.1 Jason D. Butler leading a drama therapy class at Lesley University.

Starting Out

As a young boy, my parents took the family to see a touring production of *Oliver!* at a fancy old theater in the big city. From the moment the curtain lifted, I was transfixed, completely pulled into the story. I was running the streets with Oliver, the Artful Dodger, and the rest, ready to "pick a pocket or two." The music, the sets, the lights, they all combined to transport me into another world. I was caught up in the story of Oliver Twist and the dramatic way it was performed live in front of me. From that moment, drama and theater were lifesavers for me; I truly don't know who I would be without them. After that experience, I sought out every opportunity possible to be involved with theater, on stage, backstage, handing out programs, you name it – I was hooked. Theater gave me a home, a way of expressing myself, a path to creatively collaborate with others, and the opportunity to explore new characters and ways of being in the world.

By the time I reached high school, I knew that I wanted to be a drama teacher and to help others find the magic of the stage. My father was a public school teacher, and I saw the positive impact he had on his many students. I thought that was the best way to make a difference and share my passion. Decades ago, when I was making those career decisions, I had never heard of drama therapy. At the time, the profession was relatively new and without the Internet, word of such a specialized field was not widely known. If I had been born a couple of decades later, I'm sure it would have been my first choice.

I became a high school drama teacher and thought I had found my calling. Similar to my own experience, I began noticing that the students in my classes and those who were participating in the shows were getting more out of the experiences than just learning how to be theater professionals. I watched as they made discoveries about themselves and the world through their encounters with different characters and stories. These encounters gave permission to explore new ways of being, to come out of their shell, to learn about themselves. Believing I could help more students, I completed a master's degree in Educational Counseling, thinking that I would combine the worlds of theater and counseling to more intentionally make a difference. To my shock, I discovered that "drama therapy" already existed. My future was set, and after several years of teaching in the high school, I left to become a drama therapist.

Becoming a Drama Therapy Educator

My career has taken me to many places, working with many different kinds of people. During my drama therapy graduate program, I completed an internship in a hospital with individuals who were hospitalized for severe mental illness. My second internship was working at a non-profit center that focused on helping individuals who were living on the streets of New York City and experiencing mental health concerns. I was blessed to be able to stay at that site after my graduation and continued working there for the next eight years. In that setting we would use improvisation to challenge rigid patterns of behavior and discover new ways of being in the world. We would also create plays together that explored aspects of the participants' lives and worked to transform their experience and the experience of the surrounding community. Those productions were some of the most powerful moments of theater I have ever experienced. I have worked with children in foster care, with young mothers, and in therapeutic residences for mental illness. I have also maintained a private practice where I see people looking to improve their lives and heal past traumas. I feel incredibly lucky to be able to combine both of my passions each day – theater and helping others.

For almost the past twenty years, I have also been a drama therapy educator, helping new drama therapists in their growth in the profession. Currently, I direct the drama therapy program at Lesley University in Cambridge, MA. I love watching the light and delight in my students' eyes as they discover the seemingly magical application of theater to transformation. Witnessing their connection and passion ignite as they learn the core principles and processes is powerful and consistently reaffirms my belief in the profession.

There are multiple ways of using theater to help create change. Professionally, the two categories most closely connected are drama therapy and applied theater. Applied theater is a broad category that includes forms of theater focused on shaping social change. This could include theater in education, Theatre of the Oppressed, Playback Theatre, theater for development, and some forms of prison theater. Applied theater generally emphasizes transforming society and its systems. While both applied theater and drama therapy are concerned with using drama and theater to facilitate change, drama therapy focuses more on a relationship with individual and group transformation and healing. This means drama therapists are trained as mental health practitioners who offer treatment based on the psycho-social needs of the individual or group we are working with. This training places the focus on creative therapeutic interventions that can address a wide range of conditions from trauma to schizophrenia, from autism to obsessive-compulsive disorder, from loss to just feeling stuck and unsure. As drama therapists we are prepared to work with a full spectrum of the human experience.

What about you? You've been changed by theater and drama, and you want to help other people have that same experience. What's next?! The first thing is to continue engaging with your passion and gain as much experience as possible in theater and drama while creating experiences that allow you to help others. The best foundation you can have is in the art form – any and all aspects of it, including tech theater, design, and construction. Keep feeding your passion and your creativity. These practices will continue to sustain you personally and professionally.

Educational Requirements for Drama Therapy

A master's degree is necessary in order to practice drama therapy. The North American Drama Therapy Association (NADTA), the professional association in the US and Canada, requires at least a master's degree in order to become a Registered Drama Therapist (RDT). All licenses to practice drama therapy in the States require at least a master's degree as well. While there are some introductory courses in drama therapy at the undergraduate level that you can take to become familiar with the profession, in order to become a professional drama therapist, you will need at least a master's degree.

The most common undergraduate degrees that people have previous to coming into a drama therapy program are degrees in theater and/or in psychology. These two majors provide the most solid footing for studying drama therapy. Each drama therapy graduate program requires individuals to have taken coursework in both. If you don't have an undergrad major in either of these, no need to worry. A major is not required, as long as you can show that you have coursework and experience in both areas. My pro tip is to make sure that you have as much of a foundation in theater as possible. At the undergraduate level, your job is to become a theater artist. The graduate drama therapy programs will teach you how to focus on the mental health portions of the work to prepare you for clinical practice. Usually, they do not focus on providing theater training. Familiarity with improvisation, scene work, creating plays, etc. will help you jump right into the work.

Bring your specific strengths and passions with you to graduate school. What do you love about theater and drama? I have worked with students whose passion is stage combat, role-play games, stage design, playwriting, devising, miming, and improvisation. The fantastic thing about drama therapy is that the principles of the profession can be applied to all aspects of the craft. The purpose of graduate training in drama therapy is not about teaching you specific techniques (although we certainly do teach techniques) but more about helping you gain foundational skills and ideas about how to apply the passion and knowledge of theater and drama that you already have to create change.

The drama therapy graduate programs vary in length, with most being between two and three years from beginning to end. Each program has their own specific personality and unique focus while still following the guidelines of the NADTA. Within your program, you will take courses that are focused on mental health practices – such as human development, psychopathology, counseling skills, and group therapy. These courses help create a clinical perspective that allows you to see how an individual or group are functioning and what might be getting in the way of them functioning at an even better level. You will also take courses on research – an important need in the field for showing the public that what drama therapists do works – and ethics – keeping clients emotionally and physically safe is a responsibility of all therapists.

In addition to the mental health classes, you will take classes that teach you about the application of drama therapy to facilitate transformation and growth. Each program has its own focus and nuance, but, in all of them, you will learn the application of improvisation, masks, puppets, playwrighting, and performance to drama therapy. You will learn how to see people in terms of the roles they play in their lives, how to structure a session and series of sessions, how to tell stories for therapeutic gain, and how to put together therapeutic theater performances. Drama therapists use a wide range of drama and theater interventions intentionally to work on specific treatment plans with a variety of populations.

One of my favorite things about learning drama therapy is that the majority of classes are experiential. There are no large lecture classes in drama therapy. It would be impossible to learn how be a drama therapist without actually doing drama therapy, and so drama therapy classrooms are alive with dynamic projects where you engage hands-on with the work. Students in my classes spend time creating masks and puppets to investigate the roles that they play in their lives and work at developing new and more dynamic roles. They engage in improvisation to improve their ability to be spontaneous and flexible in the face of life's curve balls. They develop performance pieces that explore aspects of their lives in front of an audience. Together we share, laugh, cry, and learn. As students take their journey toward becoming a drama therapist, each class is a new adventure of self-discovery and application to practice. Within graduate education for drama therapy, there are very few courses you will take that are not directly connected to your passion and the path to becoming a registered drama therapist.

When it comes to becoming a quality therapist, the most important factor is your ability to form strong therapeutic relationships with the people you work with. In order to do this, we must know ourselves – and we must know ourselves in relationship to the methods we use. Because of this, drama therapy education invites you to learn more about yourself so that you can use those aspects of self to help transform individuals, groups, and communities more effectively. Drama therapists work with people from different backgrounds and cultures. Because of this, a strong focus of all the programs is on understanding our own social locators and roles within various systems. You will explore how power, privilege, and oppression play out in your life, in the lives of those you may work with, and within the therapeutic relationship itself.

In addition to the coursework, drama therapy students are required to do internships with two different populations for at least 800 hours. These internships can be in a wide variety of settings. At each internship you will have a supervisor who helps guide you through the experience, who gives you feedback on your work, and who models how to be a therapist. You will also have a supervision class where you will talk with your instructor and peers about your experiences and receive feedback for improvement. With the help of your supervisors, you can try out your ideas and get professional advice along the way. Internships are a way of implementing your learning – the laboratory where you get to start practicing drama therapy and working with actual clients. One of my favorite things is watching students spread their wings and soar into the practice they have been preparing for throughout the program.

The final portion of most programs is a culminating project. These vary by school but usually involve a written thesis, a culminating performance, or both. These culminating projects give you the chance to dive deeply into a specific topic of your choosing. You can write about the integration of musical theater and substance use treatment, create a performance about your understanding of the various roles you play in social situations and how that impacts your well-being, or do an applied project at your internship to try a new idea or explore a theory. This is where you further solidify your expertise in a particular topic and potentially set a path for your future work.

Credentialing and Continuing Education

Once you graduate, you continue to be part of the larger drama therapy community. The group you studied with for your degree often becomes some of your closest friends and colleagues. Each graduate program has a network of alumni who help, inspire, and support each other and offer resources for jobs and professional advice. Additionally, as part of the NADTA, you are immediately connected with a broad network of drama therapists throughout the world. Each year the NADTA has an annual conference where drama therapists come together to share ideas, reconnect, and move the profession forward. Drama therapists continue a process of lifelong learning, always expanding our practice, learning by engaging in professional development, and staying connected to our art. Decades after my own graduation, I love seeing my former classmates at the conferences and supporting each other in our work. It is powerful to see the various paths people have taken and the stunning impact they have had on the world.

Conclusion

I suppose I am biased, but I cannot imagine a profession that could be more fulfilling and rewarding than drama therapy. As drama therapists, we get to play the roles of the Artist and the Therapist, simultaneously, to transform our world. Each time I enter into dramatic work with clients and students, I am reminded of the unique power of theater that I first encountered so many years ago. As a drama therapist, I am blessed to join the people I work with in a creative act of discovery, healing, advocacy, and transformation. If this sounds like something you would be interested in, I encourage you to continue finding out more at the NADTA website www.nadta.org, make a phone call, send an e-mail, research the programs – the profession can always use more dynamic, passionate, creative people like you.

EDUCATION IN DANCE/ MOVEMENT THERAPY

▶ by Susan D. Imus

Susan D. Imus, MA, LCPC, BC-DMT, GL-CMA, is an associate professor at Columbia College Chicago where she created the MA program in Dance/ Movement Therapy & Counseling while chairing the Department of Creative Arts Therapy for 19 years. She cofounded the Graduate Laban Certificate in Movement Analysis (GL-CMA) program in 2001 – 2019 and founded the Shannon Hardy Making Connections Suicide Prevention Program in 2002. Susan served for nine years on the Committee of Approval for the American Dance Therapy Association (ADTA) and chaired the committee from 2006 – 2009. She chaired the Education, Research, and Practice Committee of the ADTA (2012 – 2016) and earned the first annual Excellence in Education Award by the ADTA in 2006.

Dance/movement therapy is defined as the psychotherapeutic use of dance and movement to foster the body, mind, sociocultural, and spiritual integration of an individual, a couple, family, group, or community for improving health, wellness, and healing (ADTA, 2020c). Dance/movement therapists (dmts) work in a variety of settings; anywhere that mental health services are needed. A dmt's focus is primarily on movement behavior, which serves as both the means of assessment and the mode of intervention. Verbal communication is integrated with the non-verbal and is crucial to the therapeutic relationship. How does one become a dmt?

Education in dance/movement therapy (DMT) has evolved over the past sixty years. Although dance as a healing practice is one of the oldest in civilization, the modern practice began in Western society in the twentieth century. Like most professional development, education was initiated in the apprenticeship model with individuals or small groups learning at the side of a master practitioner. The master DMT practitioners became known as first generation or the modern founders in the profession and include, but are not limited to, Marian Chace, Mary Whitehouse, Trudi Schoop, Liljan Espenak, Blanche Evan, Alma Hawkins, Elizabeth Polk, and Irmgard Bartenieff (Schmais & White, 1996). Education in the twenty-first century has transformed into national and international formalized master's programs in higher education.

Educational Pathways

Two educational pathways were created by the American Dance Therapy Association (ADTA). The ADTA was organized by seventy first- and second-generation dmts (ADTA; Schmais & White, 1996) in 1966, with Marian Chace as the first president. The ADTA mission is

> To support the profession of dance/movement therapy and is *the only US organization* dedicated to the profession of dance/movement therapy. The purpose of the ADTA is to establish, maintain, and support the highest standards of professional identity and competence among dance/movement therapists by promoting education, training, practice, and research. The Association provides avenues of communication among dance/movement therapists and those working in related fields and increases public awareness of dance/movement therapy.
>
> *(ADTA, 2020a, para. 1)*

The second generation dmts organized training programs in college and university settings. Prominent in this generation were two New Yorkers, Claire Schmais and Elissa White. They established the first DMT master's program in 1971 at Hunter College of the City University of New York with grants from the National Institute of Mental Health's Experimental and Special Training Branch Division on Manpower and Training Programs and the Department of Health, Physical Education, and Dance. Debbie Thomas started an undergraduate program at The University of Wisconsin Madison in 1972 and Miriam Berger started the second graduate program at New York University in 1973. Sixteen different master's degree programs have existed at one time or another since the inception of formalized degrees at Hunter College: eight in the east, six in the west, one in the Rockies, and one in the Midwest (Faroune, 1996). Undergraduate programs exist but do not allow the graduate to practice according to the Code of Ethics and Standards of Practice established by the ADTA (2020b). A master's degree is required to practice DMT. Two doctoral programs exist in expressive arts and creative arts therapy where one can specialize in DMT.

Another pathway called Alternate Route (AR) training exists for aspiring dmts to earn the credential to practice DMT. "The Alternate Route requires a master's degree (or higher) from an accredited institution of higher learning in combination with specific general training and dance/movement therapy coursework, fieldwork experience, and a DMT internship" (Dance/Movement Therapy Certification Board, 2020, p. 13). AR courses are offered by board-certified dance/movement therapists (BC-DMTs) across the nation and internationally. There are approximately 50 different courses offered each year. The courses must be approved by the Sub-committee on the Approval of Alternate Route Courses (SAARC) of the Committee on Approval in the ADTA. As of 2021, students must work with an approved BC-DMT advisor for a minimum of two years, but coursework is self-directed. The AR student takes classes with an individual educator or with an AR Training program where a group of individual educators have come together to create a program outside of a university setting. A few university programs allow students to attend as a student-at-large to meet AR requirements. A letter of intent after earning 8 credits is required to formally begin the AR process. Coursework must be completed within 10 years. The Standards, located on the ADTA website, explain the process.

The Committee on Approval and the Education Committee of the ADTA are responsible for educational oversight in the profession. The Committee on Approval approves master's degree programs and annually ensures educational standards are followed in colleges, universities, and in AR coursework. The Education Committee updates the Standards of Education with full board approval that AR educators and approved master's degree programs must follow.

Academic Content

The academic content at Hunter College in 1971 consisted of courses in Dance Therapy and Practice, Movement Observation, Systematic Study of Movement Behavior, Anatomy and Kinesiology, and Small Group Process (Schmais & White, 1973). The course of study was 30 credits and spanned three semesters. Fifty years later, the length of study has doubled as well as the credits earned. The typical length of study is 2.5 to 3 years to earn a master's through the Approved Program (AP) pathway. Many APs have added counseling curriculum and expanded their academic content to include courses in psychopathology, human development, addiction counseling, couples and family counseling, career counseling, and counseling theories and practice, totaling 60 credits. Most of the current approved programs meet the requirements for counseling licensure in their state and include it within the degree title, i.e., Master of Arts in Dance/Movement Therapy and Counseling or Master of Arts in Clinical Mental Health Counseling with a Dance/Movement Therapy Specialization.

Although specific counseling-related courses have been listed, the current ADTA's Standards of Education and Clinical Training (Standards; ADTA, 2020d) requires learning outcomes and competencies, not specific courses. The following required content is included within the Standards: history, theory, practice, and professional development in DMT. The theoretical content that substantiates the core content of dance/movement therapy includes: Dance, Relationships, Human Development, Neuroscience, and Assessment. The Standards include operationalized competencies that exist in the following core categories:

- Elements of dance and movement in health and healing
- Creativity and aesthetics
- Psychology of groups and group process
- Dance/movement therapy group work
- Therapeutic movement relationship
- Body/mind integration
- Neurology of movement
- Neuropsychology
- Movement observation, assessment, and analysis
- Assessment tools
- Multidisciplinary psychodiagnosis (ADTA, 2020d)

Students are ensured an inclusive and diverse education by the ADTA Standards for Education and Clinical Training (Standards) in the United States. The purpose is to ensure best practices are adhered to in administration, teaching, and supervision in both approved master's degree programs and AR training.

> A globally minded and multi-culturally competent education will prepare dance/movement therapists to be leaders and practitioners who continuously strive to contribute to a more just and equitable society.
> *(ADTA, 2020d, p. 4)*

Prior to 2017, AR and AP requirements were separate. Standards provide guidance for both AR and AP educators, administrators, and supervisors. The Standards establish that,

> An integrated dance/movement therapy education… takes place in the social context of the society in which the institution is located. This social context both prescribes and challenges issues of authority and agency, race, gender identity and relationships, educational norms, definition of health, sense of self, and disclosure.
> *(ADTA, 2020d, p. 6)*

The integration in Approved Programs is therefore between the social context (culture), the clinical institution, its supervisors, the academic program, its academic institution, and the academic faculty. In the AR track, the integration is between the BC-DMT advisor, the AR educators, the clinical institutions, and its clinical and BC-DMT supervisors.

DMT educators must have earned at minimum their BC-DMT and, according to the Standards,

> …must identify with and contribute to the dance/movement therapy profession through (1) maintaining ADTA membership; (2) maintaining BC-DMT credentialing through continuing education and upholding the ADTA Code of Ethics; (3) teaching, supervision, service, research, scholarship, advocacy, and/or practice in the field of dance/movement therapy.
>
> *(ADTA, 2020d, p. 9)*

Most educators are also licensed by their state in counseling or a related mental health field. They are required to be specialists in the content in which they teach. For example, BC-DMTs teaching movement observation and assessment are usually certified movement analysts (CMA, GL-CMA or CLMA), although this is changing in the discipline, as more culturally sensitive frameworks for movement assessment are being incorporated.

Internship

Internship is crucial for skill development and practice in DMT education. A minimum of 700 hours over six months is required in a "clinical facility which is licensed, accredited, or a therapeutic setting, which provides clinical experience and in-service education" (ADTA, 2020d, p. 13). By the end of the internship, the intern is expected to be ready for practice in the field. Fieldwork precedes internship and must cover at minimum 200 hours. Two differing populations are required for clinical experience, so students are usually assigned to one clinical institution for fieldwork and one for internship. The clinical sites span settings in mental health, healthcare, education, rehabilitation, wellness, prevention, corrections, addiction, community health, disabilities, family and childhood institutes, domestic violence, senior care, and refugee care, to name a few. In the Hunter College program, the following institutions were the first formalized internships: Bronx State Hospital, Bronx, NY; the Yale Psychiatric Institute, New Haven, CT; Essex County Hospital, Cedar Grove, NJ; St. Elizabeth's Hospital, Washington, DC; and the Ashbourne School, Philadelphia, PA (Schmais & White, 1973). It is not uncommon for Approved

Programs to have over 300 clinical sites on record for students to begin their selection process. Students must interview with the sites to be accepted for their internship.

Clinical supervision is essential to internship. BC-DMT supervisors are often employed by the fieldwork or internship site where the student completes their clinical training within the clinical institution. If one is not available on site, the academic program will contract with a BC-DMT supervisor. AR students must procure a site and supervisor with assistance from their DMT advisor. A minimum of seventy hours of supervision is required to earn the R-DMT credential. Site supervisors must have at minimum a master's degree, ideally in a mental health-related field.

Preparation for Graduate Education in Approved Programs

Academic preparation

An undergraduate education in psychology and dance is a recommended combination of study for admissions into DMT graduate school. Majoring or minoring in one or the other is ideal. This is not to say that other undergraduate degrees would not be acceptable. It is essential that the interested student check the requirements for the educational institution where they are interested in applying. Each school has their own admission criteria, but all require either an in-person movement assessment or a movement video submission. A good candidate has earned a 3.0 or better in their academic grade-point. Acceptance into a graduate program is competitive.

Dance experience

It is not necessary to be a professional dancer to become a dmt. However, a good degree of proficiency in at least one, if not two, dance styles is required. Although first and second generation dmts were skilled primarily in modern dance, all dance forms are acceptable: hip hop, ballet, jazz, modern, improvisation, liturgical, ballroom, traditional/ethnic/folk—African, Caribbean, Korean, Latin, Middle Eastern, Native American, and Flamenco. The most important skills are to be comfortable in one's moving body, understand its use in movement execution, be able to verbally communicate the moving experience, and move empathically with others. Teaching, performing, and choreography experience are recommended.

Life experience

It is an advantage for a qualified candidate to have life experience as a volunteer or work experience in human services. Many students have served as camp counselors or taught dance to vulnerable populations. They may have served as a senior care health aide or worked as a mental health tech in a psychiatric clinic. Most undergraduate colleges and universities offer community engagement opportunities for students to gain life experience in diverse, inclusive, and socially minded organizations during their studies. Cultural humility is essential in studying and working in the discipline of DMT. If the candidate does not have this maturity, an admission committee may recommend that the candidate work in the community and apply again after achieving more life experience.

Life experience also includes bio-psycho-sociocultural and spiritual awareness. The Hunter College DMT program in the early 1970s included psychological interviews in their admission selection, which were conducted by experienced psychologists. The Hunter College Dance Therapy Master's Program Manual (1973) specifically illustrated the challenges in identifying personality traits that may cause difficulty for the candidate's success in the discipline. "We recognized some of the difficulties involved in screening candidates for a new discipline. For example, a number of the characteristics and qualifications we felt to be necessary, such as certain types of personality traits, are not always clearly overt" (Schmais & White, 1973, p. 4). This remains a challenge today for graduate admissions wanting to ensure a good psychological fit for those choosing a career in a mental health-related course of study. A perfect fit can never be totally ensured, but the following abilities are essential to be successful in graduate education and a DMT career: to take feedback for personal and professional growth and development, to listen, to work well with others, to lead, and to have compassion for self and others.

Credentialing and Continuing Education

The Dance/Movement Therapy Certification Board (DMTCB), developed in 2009, is a separate non-profit credentialing organization from the professional membership organization, the ADTA. The certification board awards two levels of credentialing, the registered dance/movement therapist (R-DMT) and the board-certified dance/movement therapist (BC-DMT).

> The R-DMT represents attainment of a basic level of competence, signifying both the first level of entry into the profession and the individual's

preparedness for employment as a dance/movement therapist within a clinical and/or educational setting. The Board-Certified Dance/Movement Therapist (BC-DMT) credential can be obtained after the R-DMT is awarded, with additional requirements and experience. BC-DMT is the advanced level of dance/movement therapy practice, signifying both the second level of competence for the profession and the individual's preparedness to provide training and supervision in dance/movement therapy, as well as engage in private practice.

(ADTA, 2020c)

AR students must individually compile their coursework to apply to the DMTCB to earn their first-level credential, the R-DMT. Students who attend one of the approved master's degree programs earn the R-DMT upon successful graduation and application to the ADTA. These credentials are a national registry and certification. It should be noted that credentialing is distinct from licensure.

The Dance/Movement Therapy Certification Board grants Registry and Certification to qualified applicants. These are not equivalent to licensure. Licenses must be obtained through the appropriate licensing board(s) of state governments. The DMTCB advises students and applicants to consider the requirements for licensure as a mental health practitioner in their state of residence (Dance/Movement Therapy Certification Board, 2020, p. 3).

A credentialed dmt must partake in continuing education to remain current in the discipline and maintain their credential. Fifty hours every 5 years is the requirement for R-DMT and 100 hours for BC-DMT. A new position was created in the ADTA in 2018 to initiate and implement webinars and other educational initiatives for professionals to earn continuing education. The 3-day annual international ADTA conference, webinars, and ADTA Talks are all available through the ADTA website, www.adta.org. It is recommended that interested students participate in one of the continuing education opportunities to gain a better understanding of the discipline as well as review research and the American Journal of Dance Therapy before pursuing DMT education.

Conclusion

The American Dance Therapy Association website (www.adta.org) is the best resource for anyone interested in learning about DMT. The website includes the names of the current graduate degree programs and AR courses offered throughout the nation and internationally. As previously mentioned, it is crucial to review the specific admission requirements of each institution offering DMT degrees through Approved Programs or an allied degree, if AR training is the choice. Becoming a dmt is a challenging, yet valuable learning opportunity in not only the psychotherapeutic use of dance/movement to integrate the body, mind, and spirit for health, wellness, and healing, but to learn invaluable life skills, prepare for a health-related doctorate degree, and become a fifth generation dmt.

References

American Dance Therapy Association (ADTA). (2020a). *About the American Dance Therapy Association*. ADTA. Retrieved from https://www.adta.org/about

American Dance Therapy Association (ADTA). (2020b). *The code of ethics and standards of the American Dance Therapy Association and the Dance/Movement Therapy Certification Board*. ADTA. Retrieved from https://adta.memberclicks.net/assets/docs/Code-of-the-ADTA-DMTCB-Final.pdf

American Dance Therapy Association (ADTA). (2020c). *Frequently asked questions*. ADTA. Retrieved from https://www.adta.org/faq

American Dance Therapy Association (ADTA). (2020d). *Standards for education and clinical training*. ADTA. Retrieved from https://www.adta.org/assets/docs/7.2019-Education-Standards.pdf

Dance/Movement Therapy Certification Board. (2020). *R-DMT applicant handbook*. ADTA. Retrieved from https://adta.memberclicks.net/assets/R-DMT%20Handbook_Rev2020.pdf

Faraone, C. (1996). *The rise and fall of university sponsored dance therapy programs in the United States* (Master's thesis). Hunter College of the City University of New York.

Schmais, C., & White, E. (1973). *Hunter College dance therapy master's program manual*. Hunter College of The City University of New York, NY.

Schmais, C., & White, E. (1996). Opening keynote address, 30th Annual Conference ADTA: Where, when and how it all began. *The American Journal of Dance Therapy, 18*(1), 5–26.

SO, YOU WANT TO BE A MUSIC THERAPIST

▶ by Kenneth Aigen

Kenneth Aigen, DA, LCAT, MT-BC, is an associate professor and director of the music therapy program at New York University. He has lectured internationally and authored numerous publications on Nordoff-Robbins music therapy, qualitative research, and music-centered music therapy. His books have been translated into Chinese, Korean, and Japanese, and his most recent book is *The Study of Music Therapy: Core Issues and Concepts* (Routledge). His current research is focused on the everyday uses of music by adults on the autism spectrum.

Starting Out

> Music . . . . . . therapy. Music . . . . therapy. Music . . therapy. Music therapy!

When I first heard those two words combined into a single term, it was a moment of illumination. It was the fall of 1980, and I had completed an undergraduate degree with a double-major in philosophy and psychology, followed by two years playing in a country rock band in Wisconsin. As a native New Yorker, I returned home that fall at the age of 24, unsure of what my future held as none of my interests at the time, considered individually—working with people, a career in academia, or performing—seemed to be fulfilling to me.

After a few months living at home with my parents, two things soon became apparent: (1) it was a lot more difficult to make a living as a musician in the New York City metropolitan area than it was in Madison, Wisconsin, as most musicians played for very little pay just hoping to get exposure; (2) as a consequence of (1), I needed to find a real job. I answered an advertisement for a pianist wanted as an accompanist for a theater arts group at a school for children and adolescents with emotional challenges. The job interview consisted of working with some of the kids on a song they were rehearsing for an upcoming performance.

I was not offered the position: I was told that the school wanted someone older who would commit to the job for a longer period of time, but the director liked the way I worked with the students and offered me a job as a teacher's assistant to work in the classroom. It was not the job that I came for, but it was the one that was offered, and I really did enjoy working with the kids, so I accepted the offer on the spot.

A few days later, I was at the school to process some paperwork, and I ran into the woman who was leaving the accompanist position for which I had initially applied. She was warm and friendly and told me that she was leaving to matriculate in a master's program in music therapy at New York University. That is when I heard those two magic words, and I immediately knew what I wanted to do with my life.

In many ways, that chance meeting has determined the subsequent course of my life for the last 40 years. I found the most rewarding outlet possible for my particular constellation of musicality; I have met the most courageous individuals you could imagine through my clinical work with people who have all types of cognitive, emotional, social, and physical challenges; and I have learned how to see, listen, and feel the inner core of human beings in a way such that their outer limitations disappear. It has not just been a livelihood or a vocation, but a path of self-actualization in ways that mirrored those of the clients with whom I have worked.

The Diversity of Approaches to Music Therapy

Although music therapy is a small profession considering its number of practitioners, it is a highly diverse one with applications ranging from those that are quite traditionally medical and scientific in their focus to those who are defined more by artistic, psychotherapeutic, and relational foundations and practices. So, if you are wondering what the practice of music therapy consists of, who might benefit from it, and who would make a good candidate to practice it, the answers that you receive will depend upon whom you are asking. Anyone who provides a simple, concrete answer to these questions is likely only representing their own experience, preferences, and values.

This diversity in approaches is intrinsic to the nature of music itself. Consider other professions such as speech therapy or physical therapy. The names of these professions indicate the changes sought: communication abilities in the former and motor functioning in the latter. Music therapy is different in that the name specifies the medium of interaction rather than the targeted area of change. Because its name does not define its purpose, music therapy can bear quite diverse conceptualizations of what it is that music therapists do for, and with, their clients.

The conventional wisdom is that music therapy is the use of music to achieve nonmusical, health-related goals. In this perspective, music is merely a tool used to reach the same ends that other types of therapists work toward, and music therapists provide the same types of benefits. Whether or not a client has a particularly musical experience is not relevant, and what defines music therapy is the tool of intervention, not the goal.

However, there is another way of thinking about music therapy where music is not merely a tool but a medium of experience that provides unique benefits not offered by other types of therapies. In this perspective—known as music-centered music therapy—music is considered to be a universal health resource that provides unique experiences of oneself, one's relationship to others, and one's sense of place in the world: all necessary components of being fully human. In this view, music therapy is a means for providing access to the health affordance of music for people who cannot achieve this without special assistance. In this approach, the musicality of the client's experience is absolutely necessary because it can be included as part of the goal of the work.

Approaches to music therapy that are based upon the conventional approach include behavioral music therapy and neurologic music therapy. If that tradition appeals to you, then you would likely want to locate a music therapy program consistent with those approaches. However, if you are someone who is more interested in the creative, relational, and music-based approaches, then you would want to locate a program that is more focused on psychotherapeutic applications and that lean more upon the creative practices that underlie music-centered approaches. My preference lies in this latter realm. And full disclosure demands that I acknowledge that I am the author of a text called *Music-Centered Music Therapy* (Aigen, 2005). The balance of the contents of the present chapter is grounded in the idea that the most profound thing that we can do for clients is to provide them access to their own inner sources of creativity and artistic expression because this is where the capacity for healing and self-growth originates. This is not merely an abstract preference of mine, but something grounded in many years of clinical experience in which I engaged with a wide variety of people with diverse challenges.

Education in Music Therapy

So, what advice can I provide to individuals considering entering the profession of music therapy? Well, that depends on a few factors, including the nature of your musical skills, whether or not you already have an undergraduate degree in another area, and most importantly, what type of music therapist you would like to become.

Undergraduate education in music therapy

Music therapy is unique in the US in having a large number of undergraduate programs that prepare graduates to sit for a board certification exam offered by the Certification Board for Music Therapists (CBMT). Candidates who pass the exam earn the credential Music Therapist-Board-Certified (MT-BC). Art, dance, and drama therapy only offer the opportunity for this type of credential for individuals with graduate degrees. One reason for this difference lies in the varying history of these professions: while music therapy was an outgrowth of music education, the other arts therapies originated from psychodynamic psychotherapies.

High school graduates are able to pursue an undergraduate degree in music therapy and to take the national board-certification examination after completing a degree and its associated six-month clinical internship. As many undergraduate programs are in schools, departments, colleges, and conservatories of music, it will be necessary to pass an audition on your major instrument to be admitted to one of these programs. Although specific schools differ, on average, approximately one-quarter of your coursework will be in the area of music therapy, and you will be taking coursework and engaging in the development of performance skills required of all music students and be required to pass musical juries.

However, as you know from my brief autobiographical description at the outset, this is not the route I took. In fact, not having had formal musical training in my high school years, I did not have the types of musical skills that would have enabled me to pass an audition for a music therapy degree program. In retrospect I can say that the route I took was one that best prepared me for a lifelong career working in the music-centered approach. I was a self-taught rock musician, and I can unequivocally say that the skills that I developed in this area were precisely those that I drew upon in my music therapy practice.

Graduate education in music therapy

Depending on your age, goals, experiences, and the type of music therapist that you want to be, there are a number of good reasons to pursue a master's degree in music therapy, regardless of your current age or educational background. First, music therapists are increasingly gaining the ability to earn licenses in different states, and these licenses often require a master's degree. Also, the profession is moving in the direction of requiring the master's degree for entry-level practice. And on a pragmatic level, positions that require a graduate degree generally are endowed with greater responsibility and a higher salary. Plus, in metropolitan areas where there are graduate music therapy programs—such as Boston, Philadelphia, and New York City—positions generally require a graduate degree.

There are two additional reasons why I would recommend this route: First, if your musical identity is primarily as an instrumentalist or vocalist with advanced skills in the Western classical music tradition, it is a fact that most of what you learn and study in an undergraduate music degree will not be relevant in your music therapy practice. Music therapists are required to gain and demonstrate basic competencies on guitar, piano, and voice: the ability to play and sing basic pop songs from the last 70 years in a fluid, pleasing, musical way is far more important than are advanced skills on orchestral instruments. In preparing for a music therapy career, you would be much better off spending your time honing your piano, guitar, and vocal skills than in advancing your primary instrument skills. Consequently, any other undergraduate major, such as psychology or sociology—just to name two—will likely give you a broad-based, well-rounded educational experience that will be important in becoming the type of person who can serve as a therapist for individuals from a wide variety of age groups, ability levels, and cultures.

Second, if you are drawn more to the music-centered, psychotherapeutic, and arts-based approaches, then the graduate degree would provide you with the necessary time for the growth and maturation required for practice in these areas. If you believe in the transformative capacities of music and want to employ them to help clients effect fundamental change in their lives, you will require the support and guidance afforded by graduate degree programs.

In considering a music therapy master's degree, you will fit into one of three categories, and the options for study will vary greatly depending upon the nature of your undergraduate degree. Therefore, it is absolutely essential for you to understand the differing opportunities, whether you are reading this chapter already having completed an undergraduate degree or if you have not yet done so. Moreover, many academic music therapists are not aware of these subtle distinctions, and you may get inaccurate or incomplete guidance depending on whom you speak with. The balance of this chapter considers the opportunities for graduate study for (a) individuals with an undergraduate music therapy degree; (b) individuals with an undergraduate music degree in an area other than music therapy; and (c) individuals with an undergraduate degree in any area other than music.

Which is better? An undergraduate or a graduate degree?

For those of you who decide to earn an undergraduate degree in music therapy prior to pursuing a music therapy master's degree, you will have a great deal of choice in the number of programs as you will be eligible for any master's program. However, there is a real difference among the master's programs that you should be aware of. Most of these programs are more oriented toward acquiring research skills, and they lack a coherent conceptualization of the advanced level of clinical practice that a graduate degree should prepare you for. Therefore, I strongly encourage you to inquire about the extent to which coursework in the degree program is devoted to advanced levels of clinical practice.

These same considerations are also relevant to those of you who pursue an undergraduate degree in music prior to engaging in a music therapy master's degree program. However, there is an additional concern here that is of primary importance. You may be required to fulfill the undergraduate music therapy requirements either prior to, or concomitant with, your graduate studies. In other words, you will be asked to take undergraduate coursework together with undergraduate students as part of your degree. In effect, you will be earning an undergraduate equivalency degree as a prerequisite for your graduate music therapy studies. And again, you should determine if there is dedicated graduate level coursework oriented toward advanced levels of clinical practice or if most of the master's study is research-oriented, which will leave you with entry-level clinical skills.

And last, for readers who possess an undergraduate degree in a nonmusical area, there are only a few options for you. Lesley University, Drexel University, and New York University (full disclosure: I am the director of the NYU program), are the only schools that I am aware of that allow students to matriculate directly into a master's level music therapy program without an undergraduate music degree. This option has many advantages that I will detail below, but it is a fact that many music therapy educators are not aware of this option. Thus, it is possible that you have not heard of this possibility or that you have been given incorrect information about it.

You might be wondering why such an important option is so rarely offered and not widely known. Without going into too much detail, I would like to provide some historical background on this issue. For 28 years, from 1970 through 1998, there were two music therapy associations in the US: the American Association for Music Therapy (AAMT) and the National Association for Music Therapy (NAMT). The former organization was located primarily in the northeast and was significantly smaller than the latter organization. Although smaller, the AAMT was more devoted to graduate education as the minimum standard for clinical practice. When the two organizations unified in 1998 (under the name American Music Therapy Association), both education and training models were accepted, but most educators in the larger association remained unaware of the educational policies of the smaller one. (For a first-hand account of the unification process, see Aigen and Hunter, 2018.)

There are a number of reasons why the structure of educational programs such as those at Drexel, Lesley, and NYU offer advantages to students. (1) All of the coursework is at the graduate level, which means that, even when introductory material is being covered, it will be addressed at a graduate level of sophistication. (2) These graduate programs are more diverse in terms of age, cultural background, musical identities, and life experience of their students. There is more to be gained educationally from a cohort that has more diversity within it, especially in programs that emphasize the self-growth aspects of becoming a therapist. (3) Entry-level master's programs tend to have a much better integration of classroom experience and clinical experience. Although they offer pre-internship experiences along with coursework, most undergraduate programs in music therapy are structured in a way where the largest amount of clinical experience (the formal internship) takes place after coursework is completed. In contrast, at a program such as NYU, students are placed in a clinical setting from their first week in the program through the last week. The school closely monitors the internship and is in constant contact with the internship supervisor, while the student attends a supervision seminar at the school along with other students in their internship placement. This arrangement greatly enhances cooperation between the school and the clinical site, something that works to the student's advantage. (4) Music therapists are becoming eligible for licensure in an increasing number of states. These licenses generally require a master's degree with a certain number of minimum credits. In earning a master's degree, a student enters the profession better prepared for an extended career.

I would like to make one caveat here: governmental and educational standards are always changing. There is no way to know for how long the information I have provided to you in this essay will remain accurate. Therefore, it is essential that you verify these items when you are making your decision about pursuing a music therapy degree.

Conclusion

Music therapists are artists that use music to promote the well-being and quality of life of their clients. Some think of themselves as therapists who use music as a tool; others consider themselves first and foremost as musicians who work for the health of the individuals and communities with whom they are engaged; and still others, fully embrace the *sui generis* category of music therapist as someone who exists apart from any other conventional social category. In my career and life as a music therapist, I have met colleagues from all these different orientations. I hope that this profession continues to be one where these differences can coexist, because this is the best way to ensure that it can offer the diversity of services demanded by the diversity of clients who are engaged in it.

References

Aigen, K. (2005). *Music-centered music therapy*. Barcelona.

Aigen, K. (2014). *The study of music therapy: Current issues and concepts*. Routledge.

Aigen, K., & Hunter, B. (2018). The creation of the American Music Therapy Association: Two personal perspectives. *Music Therapy Perspectives, 36*(2), 183–194.

EDUCATION AS AN ART THERAPIST

▶ by Gaelynn Wolf Bordonaro

Gaelynn Wolf Bordonaro, Ph.D., ATR-BC, is the director of the Graduate Art Therapy Program at Emporia State University in Emporia, KS and a Roe R. Cross distinguished professor in the department of Counselor Education. She has also taught art therapy courses at Florida State University, University of Louisville, and La Trobe University (Melbourne, Australia). Wolf Bordonaro serves on the Art Therapy Credentials Board (ATCB) and is the clinical director of Communities Healing through Art (CHART), and she served four terms on the board of directors of the American Art Therapy Association (AATA). She is particularly interested in international art therapy trauma response programming, pediatric and palliative medical art therapy, and the use of photography and art therapy with children with medical and physical disabilities; she has presented on art therapy topics on six continents and throughout the United States.

It is a pleasure to share information and strategies as you consider or pursue a career in the creative arts therapies. In fact, many of the contributors to this text may wish this type of resource existed when we first learned about our fields! I'm happy to share my perspectives as the director of the Emporia State University Art Therapy Program in Emporia, Kansas.

More than 30 universities in the United States offer graduate art therapy programs. The oldest art therapy programs were established in the late 1960s and early 1970s, and most of the programs have been preparing exceptional art therapists for decades! The field of art therapy is relatively close knit, and art therapy educators from the diverse universities have often enjoyed opportunities to work together on national boards, committees, research, publications, curriculum design, and projects; art therapy educators are also outstanding art therapy clinicians, researchers, advocates, and authors. They are also well-connected to exceptional practitioners throughout the field and can provide wonderful networking opportunities for students. The bulk of art therapy graduate programs are housed in private universities, but four public universities have long-running graduate therapy programs (Emporia State University in Emporia, KS; Florida State University in Tallahassee, FL; Southern Illinois University in Edwardsville, IL; and the University of Louisville, KY).

A Quick Discussion about Program Accreditation

The website of the American Art Therapy Association (AATA) has links to art therapy graduate programs accredited by the Commission on Accreditation of Allied Health Education Programs, managed through the Accreditation Council for Art Therapy Education (CAAHEP/ACATE). Accreditation indicates the program has undergone an extensive and on-going external quality review. The educational standards for accredited art therapy programs can be found online (CAAHEP/ACATE, CAAHEP Standards Template II). Identifying programs accredited by CAAHEP/ACATE can be a very important step for students, as it can directly impact credentialing and state licensure processes in states that have art therapy licenses after students have completed their master's degree.

The Art Therapy Credentials Board (ATCB) was founded in 1993 to protect the public by promoting the competent and ethical practice of art therapy (atcb.org). It is the agency that manages the credentialing and testing processes of art therapists to ensure the professional, ethical, high-quality practice of the profession. Graduates of CAAHEP-accredited art therapy programs are required to complete a minimum of 1,000 post-graduate, direct client contact hours using art therapy before applying for the Registered Art Therapist (ATR) credential. Graduates of art therapy programs that are not accredited are required to complete 1,500 hours of post-graduate direct client contact hours before applying for the ATR.

Applying for Art Therapy Graduate Study

To apply for graduate programs, a student must have earned a bachelor's degree. Many students who apply to graduate programs have pursued undergraduate majors and/or minors in disciplines related to art therapy (i.e., art, psychology, sociology, or education); however, students with other areas of concentration should not be discouraged from applying. I had the honor of chairing a master's thesis committee for an exceptional art therapy scholar, Seungbin Oh (2015), whose undergraduate degree was in accounting! His background had prepared him well for the data collection and analysis needed for art therapy research.

A number of universities and colleges offer pre-art therapy majors or minors. It is important to remember that these programs are not the only path to graduate study in art therapy, and they are not designed to prepare students to practice art therapy. Neither a BA nor a BS in Art Therapy will qualify you to practice art therapy; a master's degree is required. Some programs offer non-clinical (*not* therapy) brief internship experiences. Some are designed and directed by art therapists with art therapists teaching core courses. Others are simply designed to make sure students complete all the prerequisites needed for graduate study in art therapy. Either emphasis is fine.

The title of the undergraduate degree is generally not as important as having earned the bachelor's degree and having completed the prerequisites for the universities to which you will apply. Those prerequisites can vary, but often they include a specific number of credit hours in psychology coursework and a specific number of credits in studio art. For example, many graduate programs require 12 credit hours of psychology (to include Abnormal Psychology and Developmental Psychology), and 18 credit hours of studio art. Importantly, art history and art appreciation courses don't count. The studio art courses may include drawing, painting, sculpture, photography, graphic arts, 2D design, 3D design, fibers and fabrics, jewelry making, glass forming, and more. Be sure to check program websites to be certain if specific courses, such as drawing and painting, are required.

If you are in contact with a faculty member or program representative from the program(s) to which you will apply, they are often happy to take a look at your unofficial transcripts and unofficially let you know if you have deficits in your prerequisites. It's a good idea to initiate contact before your senior year of your undergrad program, so if you still need courses that are required by the graduate program, you will have time to fit them in your program of study. If you graduated from college a number of years before applying to graduate school, check with the program director as well.

Application Requirements

Perhaps the most intimidating part of a graduate school application is the personal essay. This may take the form of a cover letter, or it may be in response to questions on the application. Create your narrative in a separate document before cutting and pasting into the application. Read and reread the narrative, then ask a colleague, academic advisor, or better yet, someone from the Career Services Office at your undergraduate university to review it. Even if you have already graduated, most Career Services Offices are happy to provide feedback on your applications for graduate school. If an interview is required or requested, the Career Services Office may even offer mock interviews to polish your interview skills.

Art therapy graduate applications require a portfolio. Often, 15 – 20 pieces are required. Be sure to include the number of images the university specifies. Although some programs may ask for other formats, often PowerPoint is the format of choice and can be easily uploaded to universities' application sites. Make sure photos or scans of your work are clear and cropped so the full image can be seen. Include a title or indicate if the work is untitled, the year it was completed, and the media used. Brief artist statements may be required, but even if they are not, they are welcomed. If you are photographing a 3D piece, large or small, pay close attention to the background to reduce distractions or provide context.

Letters of recommendation are rich sources of information for application review committees. Whether the university has a form for your references to complete or requires a submitted letter, thoughtful narratives are helpful! If Likert Scale items are on a form that is to be completed, ask your reference to include examples of your strengths, rather than just picking a number on a scale of 1 – 5. Examples of leadership in the classroom, special projects, research initiated, or even instances of successful problem-solving can help an application review committee understand how you will perform in graduate school. Psychology and art faculty are ideal people to ask for recommendations (at least one of each, if possible). A work supervisor can be appropriate too, particularly if the work emphasized interpersonal relationships (i.e., teaching or tutoring, childcare or nursing care, serving as a camp counselor, or working with individuals with disabilities). Applicants who have been out of school for a long period of time may need to rely on references from work supervisors if they have not been in contact with their professors. Unless an application explicitly requests a personal reference, do *not* submit recommendations from relatives or friends.

Some universities may require applicants to take the Graduate Record Examination (GRE), but this is not as common as it was just a few years ago. The GRE helps review committees determine applicants' qualifications and preparedness for graduate-level study; scores are used to assess readiness to succeed in a rigorous course of study. If a program to which you are applying requires the GRE, you can find venues in your community which offer the computer-based, standardized exam. Scores will be reported directly to the universities you indicate.

An official transcript will be required as part of your application. The Records Office or Registrar's Office at your undergraduate university will send an official transcript to the graduate school for a nominal fee.

Tips for Applications/Applicants

Unlike portfolios for a Master of Fine Arts (MFA) application, art therapy programs seek students who are familiar with diverse media and are able to use them expressively. Rather than a portfolio emphasizing mastery of a single media and exceptional technique with that media, application reviewers value prospective students' demonstration of basic skills and creativity with multiple art media, and even non-traditional media. Of course, portfolios can include technically exceptional work, but they shouldn't be limited to those pieces. If you love a piece of artwork you created because it captures a mood or a favorite moment, most programs would welcome a brief narrative in the portfolio that explains why you connect with the piece, even though it's not a masterpiece.

If you are thinking ahead to graduate school, it is a great idea to find opportunities to work or volunteer in roles that use art with others. Many communities have camps for children or teens with specials needs, rehabilitation centers may offer workshops or arts classes, and community pop-up studios are growing in popularity. Planning and initiating art experiences, building on the skills and interests of participants, and observing the different ways that people engage with art materials are valuable introductions to a career in the expressive arts. Additionally, hands-on engagement provides meaningful experiences about which you can write in your personal essay.

Preparing for Training in a Helping Profession

Art therapy is a human service profession. A rich foundation in psychology and studio art are important parts of your preparation. However, interpersonal skills and intrapersonal development are essential as well. Friends may describe you as a good listener or as open-minded. Professors or supervisors may have commented on your critical thinking skills or your ability to work well as part of a team. These characteristics suggest you are on the right path. However, in addition to personality traits and behavioral qualities, there are things you can actively do to prepare yourself for a rewarding career that marries the worlds of art and service to others.

For anyone who plans to be a mental health professional, I highly recommend the experience of engaging in therapy. If you haven't already, find a therapist and get started. Students can take advantage of free or very low cost services through campus wellness centers. In addition to counselors and social workers, a limited number of college campuses have art therapists available, and many art therapists work in private practice or in agencies that serve the local community. Invest in the opportunity to process difficult experiences, tackle personal concerns, and confront stigma associated with mental health treatment directly by participating in the work of therapy. Helpful resources for finding a therapist who is right for you are a click away (Morin, 2020).

If you are currently a student, actively engage in campus and community-based opportunities to learn about diversity, equity, and inclusion (DEI). Even if you are not currently a student, many universities offer lectures, workshops, and trainings that will plant the seeds for your future work with people with diverse backgrounds and with diverse personal and cultural identities. Learn to acknowledge and value difference and explore your own and the broad range of lived experiences. Enjoy the hard work and learning that shape advocacy, anti-racism, and exceptional art therapists; the learning and the journey never stop.

You Have Been Accepted! What's Next?

I have wonderful professional and personal relationships with art therapy educators across the nation and even in other countries. One of the things I often hear from faculty members is that students are not prepared to write at the graduate level. Some students feel confident in their creative writing abilities but struggle with academic writing. Many are only peripherally familiar with the writing standards of the American Psychological Association (also known as APA style). If it's been a while since you took a composition course, or you struggle with grammar, clarity, or organization in your writing, consider opportunities to brush up on your writing skills. Abbreviated courses can be found online, and many can be audited without charge. If you plan to start your graduate program at the beginning of the fall semester, the summer may be a perfect time to invest in your academic writing skills; the investment will pay dividends your very first semester and beyond! Purchase the most recent edition of the APA Manual and begin to review it before your first semester starts. Once you settle into your campus community, be sure to find the writing center on your campus and connect with the amazing librarians in your university's library.

If you have a learning disability or require any type of accommodation, make an appointment to talk with or meet the staff of the Accessibility Services Office at your new university. Part of becoming a competent professional mental health services provider is recognizing your personal strengths and challenges. Don't wait to self-advocate. Accessibility is about making sure that *everyone* can partake in the many rich experiences graduate school and the broader world can offer.

Your art therapy program will likely have a student association that welcomes graduates and undergraduates pursuing a career in art therapy. Learn when they meet and get involved. Some student art therapy organizations/associations/clubs focus on fund-raising to help members attend state and national conferences; in fact, most universities' student government associations provide funding support to recognized student organizations' participation in professional development activities, such as conferences and hosting speakers. Other art therapy student organizations highlight community and campus service through the arts. Some organizations are dedicated to social justice and anti-racism education and diversity, equity, and inclusion advocacy. Others provide opportunities for group art-making and self-care. Many art therapy student groups combine these important areas of interest. It's worth noting that the leaders of these groups, generally elected by their members, play considerable roles in shaping the vision for the group for the year of their elected position; if you are passionate about advocacy, self-care, service, or another application of the arts in society, do seriously consider a leadership role as part of your academic career.

Finally, practice what you preach! In your personal essay in application for graduate study of art therapy, you may have shared your own experiences with the centering, restorative, and stress-reducing qualities of art-making. The assignment deadlines, academic expectations, time-management requirements, multi-tasking demands, and other pressures experienced by graduate students can be downright stressful. If art-making transports you to your happy place, do it! Importantly, don't just think longingly about making art; you will likely need to purposely schedule it into your week, and then commit to it. Make it part of your self-care routine, just like getting enough sleep, eating plenty of fruits and vegetables, and connecting with important people in your life.

References

Oh, S. (2015). *The cross-cultural utility of the formal elements of art therapy scale and the person picking an apple from a tree.* Unpublished Master's Thesis, Emporia State University, Emporia, KS.

Morin, A. (2020). How to choose the right therapist for you. Retrieved from https://www.ver ywellmind.com/how-to-choose-the-right-therapist-for-you-4842306

WRITE ON! POETRY THERAPY, JOURNAL THERAPY, AND TRANSFORMATIVE LANGUAGE ARTS

▶ by Kathleen Adams

Kathleen Adams LPC, PTR, is a licensed therapist and registered poetry/journal therapist who has pioneered the field of journal therapy since 1985. She is the author of 13 books on writing for healing, growth, and change, including the best-selling classic *Journal to the Self* (1990), the text *Expressive Writing: Foundations of Practice* (2013), and *Journal Therapy for Calming Anxiety* (2020). She is a three-time recipient of the National Association for Poetry Therapy's Distinguished Service Award and has also received NAPT's Morris Morrison Education Award for excellence in training and professional education. Kathleen is the founder/director of the Center for Journal Therapy (1988), the Therapeutic Writing Institute (2008), and Journalversity (2017).

How many of these statements are true for you?

- ☐ You've loved stories since you were a child.
- ☐ You have a creative imagination.
- ☐ English was one of your favorite subjects.
- ☐ You like to work or study in small groups or classes.
- ☐ You've always wanted to write a book.
- ☐ You love the way some song lyrics or poems make you feel.
- ☐ You write poetry or song lyrics of your own.
- ☐ You have a gift for helping others.
- ☐ You want a career that allows you to help people grow and change.
- ☐ You love the visual storytelling of movies and TV series.
- ☐ You have written a journal at some point in your life, and it has been useful in helping you solve problems and discover more about yourself.
- ☐ You identify with fictional characters and use them as role models to help you think through your own experiences or solve your own problems.

☐   Writing, reading, or listening to songs, poems, journal entries, short stories, etc. makes you feel better (or smarter, clearer, stronger, calmer, etc.)

If you checked some of these boxes – there may be a career in applied poetry or journal facilitation in your future!

Writing and Literature As Pathways to Healing

The recognition of poetry and writing as holistic wellness tools has never been higher. Many health and wellness programs, recovery methods, spiritual practices, psychotherapy models, management experts, and self-help authors recommend some method of life documentation as a primary path to well-being and self-management.

Social science research shows that writing about difficult experiences can create pathways to health. Therapists, counselors, and coaches recommend writing to clients as a way of accelerating positive change. Community facilitators create writing circles where people in pain find comfort and clarity.

The purposeful and intentional use of written and spoken language to effect growth and positive change – variously called expressive writing, therapeutic writing, poetry therapy, journal therapy, or transformative language arts (TLA) – is an accessible and easy-to-use tool for holistic mental, emotional, physical, and spiritual well-being.

Since the mid-20th century, poetry therapy, journal therapy, and TLA have been at the forefront of this shift toward public awareness of the healing power of literature and the written and spoken word. Now the fields are proud standard bearers for education, training and credentialing, creating new generations of practitioners, facilitators, community teachers, thinkers, and leaders.

About the "T-word"

Although the fields are called poetry therapy or journal therapy, the practice of actual therapy is done only by licensed therapists. As a facilitator-in-training, you will learn how to hold the boundary so that you are working at the developmental level, which means that you will provide quality psychoeducation and process around the "everyday normal" situations that happen across the life span. The release of stress and the actualization of personal growth in many different areas are the province of the certified applied poetry or journal facilitator.

Poetry Therapy

The term "poetry therapy" globally encompasses interactive bibliotherapy, journal therapy, therapeutic storytelling, as well as performance poetry. However, poetry therapy is also a defined segment of this collective, as is journal therapy. These two modalities will be discussed separately from the collective.

The field of poetry therapy as we currently know it was created in the 1970s when Dr. Jack Leedy, a New York City psychiatrist, and Dr. Art Lerner, a Los Angeles psychologist, combined their separate theories and approaches to found an organization, the National Association for Poetry Therapy, to promote education and standards-based practice in the field.

They were soon joined by Sr. Arleen Hynes in Washington DC, the librarian for St. Elizabeth's Hospital, the oldest federal in-patient psychiatric hospital in the United States. Hynes convened patient groups and offered literary selections to meet goals such as improving the capacity to respond, experiencing the liberating quality of beauty, increasing self-understanding, and clarifying personal relationships. She called this work bibliotherapy. The poetry therapy field later adopted Hynes' stated goals as its own.

As its own discipline, poetry therapy uses literature, predominantly contemporary poetry, as a catalyst for the healing process. It promotes growth and healing through the reading and facilitated discussion of literary material.

The certified or registered poetry therapist (CPT or PTR), or the certified applied poetry facilitator (CAPF), work in community centers, schools, hospitals, rehabilitation centers, prisons, places of worship, and many other aspects of community life.

Becoming a certified or registered poetry therapist
Either of these tracks require at least a master's degree in counseling or social work, as well as licensure from the state in which services are delivered.

Becoming a certified applied poetry facilitator

This is the developmental track, which can be pursued with a bachelor's degree in any field. Although the most common fields are liberal arts and social sciences, there is no restriction. Highly successful CAPFs have had undergraduate degrees in areas as far-flung as chemistry or mechanical engineering.

Assuming you are not planning on first becoming a therapist and then taking specialized training, you can become credentialed as a certified applied poetry facilitator (CAPF) through the guided independent study program of the International Federation for Biblio/Poetry Therapy (IFBPT, or "the Federation"). The Federation is the standards-setting and credentialing board for the therapeutic writing community.

The CAPF is earned through completion of 440 hours of work divided among four areas: Didactic learning such as coursework, reading, and annotating primary texts in the field, seminars and conferences (200 hours); experiential learning through participating in facilitated poetry therapy groups (60 hours); fieldwork in which trainees conduct their own poetry therapy groups (120 hours); and supervision with a Federation-approved mentor/supervisor (60 hours). The typical program takes two to three years to complete, although the Federation allows up to five years for completion.

The relationship with the mentor/supervisor (M/S) is established before training begins. A CAPF candidate chooses a mentor/supervisor from among experienced poetry therapists or facilitators who have at least two years of fieldwork and have undergone a supervisory internship with an experienced M/S.

The mentor/supervisor assists in preparing the training application to the Federation and guides the trainee through all stages of learning, including providing oversight of the facilitation planning, development, and execution. The mentor/supervisor also supports the CAPF trainee in learning from the facilitation experiences by carefully deconstructing sessions to celebrate the places of strength and to examine the places of challenge or difficulty.

More information about the Federation and the CAPF program can be found at www.ifbpt.org.

Journal Therapy

Journal therapy is the purposeful and intentional use of life-based writing to further mental, physical, emotional, and spiritual health and wellness. It offers an effective means of providing focus and clarity to issues, concerns, conflicts, and confusions. In practice, it is the act of writing down thoughts and feelings to sort through problems and come to deeper understandings of yourself or the issues in your life.

Unlike traditional diary writing, where daily events and happenings are recorded from an exterior point of view, journal therapy focuses on your internal experiences, reactions, and perceptions. Through this act of literally reading your own mind, you are able to perceive experiences more clearly and thus reduce stress and tension. Research shows this has both mental and physical health benefits.

Journal therapy came into popular use after Dr. Ira Progoff, a New York City depth psychologist and researcher, made his Intensive Journal® method available to the public in 1966. The Progoff method is profound, yet it is hampered by the amount of time and focus it takes to achieve the depth dimension.

In the mid-1980s, Dr. James Pennebaker, a research psychologist in Texas, began publishing his findings on writing as a tool for emotional and physiological stress release. Results were consistent after only four 15 – 20-minute episodes of structured writing, spaced one day apart. Pennebaker's method quickly became the standard for other researchers, and 35 years later, there is ample evidence that writing does, in fact, effect positive change in the writer under circumstances as varied as wound-healing after surgery or management of chronic long-term mental health or physical illness.

Journal therapy has been used effectively for grief and loss; coping with life-threatening or chronic illness; recovery from addictions, eating disorders and trauma; improving relationships; increasing communication skills; developing healthier self-esteem; getting a better perspective on life; and clarifying life goals.

There are opportunities in every community to teach journal writing classes and lead therapeutic writing groups – in churches/temples/mosques, libraries, recreation centers, universities and colleges, adult education programs, clinics, corporations, employee assistance programs, psychotherapy and coaching practices, hospitals… even living rooms!

The Therapeutic Writing Institute

The Therapeutic Writing Institute (TWI), which I founded in 1988, is an online professional training program in journal therapy or journal facilitation that takes about three years to complete. It was developed as an alternative training model to the Federation's guided independent study program. TWI trainees learn to responsibly and ethically facilitate writing groups in their own communities, grounded in evidence-based theory and standards-based practice.

The Therapeutic Writing Institute training is a comprehensive program of core theory, professional development, psychological awareness, and supervised practice, taught in 8-week quarters. All learning takes place online, in an asynchronous (24/7/365) learning platform. Trainees study with an international, intentional community of caring, supportive peers where everyone is both teacher and student. All TWI classes are limited to 12 students. The average class size is seven students with a faculty member who is a specialist in the course content.

The program consists of 15 classes, seven of which are in therapeutic writing (three required core theory courses, plus four electives). Five courses in the professional development area include required coursework in marketing, curriculum development and ethics, plus two electives. The remaining three courses are a required psychological awareness series (facilitation skills, group process skills, and psychology of differences [a holistic approach to what other programs call abnormal psychology]).

As with the Federation's poetry therapy certification, supervised facilitation is also required, although measurement is in units of facilitation rather than hours clocked. A capstone project that synthesizes learning and represents a publishable white paper, book chapter, or other contribution to the body of knowledge completes the program.

Becoming a certified journal therapist

As with the Federation program, this level is reserved for those who are already licensed as therapists in the state in which they practice. The program itself is identical, with the removal of the psychological awareness series, as these areas are covered in clinical training.

Additional information about the Therapeutic Writing Institute is found at www.TWInstitute.net.

Relationship between TWI and the Federation

The International Federation for Biblio/Poetry Therapy, founded in 1981, creates and maintains standards for training and practice in the fields of biblio/poetry/journal therapy. It is the only independent, not-for-profit credentialing agency in the field.

The TWI credential attests that you have satisfactorily completed a course of study with a for-profit, leader-driven organization. The certification is only as credible as the organization granting it. In other words, because the entity granting your certification and the entity to whom you are paying money for training are one and the same, there is no inherent guarantee of objectivity, quality, or transparency.

TWI has an excellent worldwide reputation for high standards of quality, integrity, responsibility, and scholastic/professional achievement; however, even the highest quality certification is not the same as an independent credential from a standards-setting agency.

In 2012, the Therapeutic Writing Institute was honored to become the first program to be fully endorsed by the Federation as an equivalent learning method to the IFBPT's guided independent study credentialing program. Additionally, the Federation and TWI have arrived at an agreement that any graduate of either program who wishes to cross-train in the other discipline may transfer in 50% of training hours and fast-track the second certification.

Transformative Language Arts

Transformative language arts blends storytelling, drama, music, poetry, writing and performance art to build communities, restore culture and ecology, advocate for social justice, and liberate the human spirit. Its artists, scholars, and facilitators work cross-culturally to bring mentoring and advocacy through diverse language arts modalities.

Essentially rooted in oral storytelling cultures, transformative language arts is committed to bringing ancient forms of community learning to contemporary issues, whether that be racial injustice, income inequality, generational divides, climate change, unfair practices from governmental or corporate leaders, or other issues of social and global urgency. Because transformative language arts can bridge any of the creative arts therapies, it is uniquely diverse in its delivery and outcomes.

The TLA Network offers a certificate program in Transformative Language Arts Fundamentals. This program does not prepare one as a working transformative language artist. Rather, it provides a theoretical and experiential foundation. It is an excellent complement to other community-based preparation, such as a facilitator training program. Additional information can be found at www.TLANetwork.org.

Conclusion

After more than 35 years in the career field of journal and poetry therapy, I am convinced that those who are attracted to this work are among the most generous, caring, unique, funny, literate, and powerful people I have been privileged to know. Every day I wake up filled with gratitude for the opportunity to do work that matters. Then I get out of bed and get busy.

If your deep desire is to make a living doing work that you love, with clients who will surprise, delight, and inspire you with the simple brilliance of their self-expression, and colleagues who are authentically passionate about words and their healing power – then we welcome you to the world of poetry, journals, and transformative language arts. You are the future of the profession!

ENTERING A CAREER IN EXPRESSIVE ARTS THERAPY

▶ by Danielle Drake

Danielle Drake, PhD, is associate professor, program chair, and alum of the Counseling Psychology, Expressive Arts Therapy MA program at the California Institute of Integral Studies. She received her PhD in Clinical Psychology from Fielding Graduate University with her dissertation study focused on the use creativity and spirituality among African Americans, in which she developed and conducted an initial validation of the Black Spiritual Creativity Scale. Her clinical work as an expressive arts therapist engages clients in creative writing, music, and visual arts processes, where she uses a liberatory informed approach that incorporates Womanist and Black/African-centered psychologies with Narrative Therapy, Emotion Focused Therapy, and contemplative practices.

What Is Expressive Arts Therapy?

A career in expressive arts therapy can be an exciting and rewarding choice. As a professor of Expressive Arts Therapy, I often run into students who have a natural inclination toward arts-based careers but feel it an impractical choice. This idea of impracticality is often fueled by the "starving artist" image which stigmatizes and undervalues creative contributions in society. Additionally, artists often have highly attuned empathic sensibilities which can also be stigmatized as being too emotional or sensitive – believe me, I have heard it all, given my own empathic nature. What I did not realize in my younger years while selecting a career path was that these artistic and empathic gifts can be combined to create a vibrant and meaningful career within the field of psychotherapy. So, what exactly is expressive arts therapy?

Expressive arts therapists utilize the power of all of the primary arts modalities (e.g., visual arts, dance, music, poetry, drama, etc.) to create healing and transformative therapeutic experiences with clients, patients, and communities in psychotherapeutic settings. Most people understand psychotherapy to be a talk-based form of accessing mental health and wellness. Expressive arts therapists assume that there are multiple ways people communicate, talking being just one of those forms. In fact, learning styles research recognizes that individuals often use a range of learning and communication styles, including verbal, auditory, somatic, kinesthetic, etc. (Pashler, McDaniel, Rohrer, & Bjork, 2008). So rather than solely relying on verbal communication, expressive arts therapists work with their clients through a variety of well selected arts modalities, weaving the different arts within the therapeutic session, to assist clients/communities in expressing their needs and accessing unique and impactful mental health outcomes.

In this essay I will discuss 1) a brief history of the expressive arts therapy field; 2) why one might consider a career in expressive arts therapy; 3) basic qualifications to enter an expressive arts therapy training program; 4) the learning involved in an expressive arts therapy training and education; 5) the additional practicum, internship, or post-graduate requirements necessary; and 6) the types of registrations and designations available within an expressive arts therapy career.

History of the Expressive Arts Therapy Field

The history of expressive arts goes back as far as the first humans living in community together. At its foundation, expressive arts is rooted in communal creative ceremony and ritual. The earliest societies wove together music, drumming, dancing, body adornment, ritual, food, song, storytelling, etc. to mark particular rites of passage. As such, expressive arts are inherently indigenous and have represented the people, places, cultures, and ethnicities engaging in it. The formalized field of expressive arts therapy came about in the 1970s through work among Paulo Knill, Shaun McNiff, Stephen Levine, Natalie Rogers, Helen Nienhaus Barba, Margo Fuch, among many others (Knill, Nienhaus, Barba, & Fuchs, 2004). In March 1974, the Institute for the Arts and Human Development at Lesley College in Cambridge, Massachusetts, became the first educational institute to develop and offer a master's program focused on creative arts therapy.

It was here that the focus on achieving depth through breadth, that is, engaging a depthful process through weaving the wide array of all forms of creative expression, was articulated in a creative arts therapy academic training program. The philosophy of the training program supported the ideas of total expression and the cultivation of sacred presence (Knill et al., 2004). Expressive arts therapy as a formalized field continues to root itself in the idea that engaging mindful and intentional presence, building one art process layered into and onto another, makes each expression more vital to the process, and each art form more inseparable from the next.

Why Expressive Arts Therapy?

Expressive arts therapy can make the sometimes daunting task of talk therapy more palatable for people whose primary response style is less verbal. Clients challenged by the verbal demands of talk therapy can have alternative response styles. A client can warm into a session using music from a playlist, an impromptu drawing, a sound, or movement/gesture. Accessing a non-verbal response alternative first can open up the pathway for verbal communication. It can also aid in the development of the therapeutic relationship between client and therapist by creating a safe, warm, and often enjoyable environment. Playfulness and humor, often woven into expressive arts therapeutic interventions, can soften the edges of the difficult life experiences and narratives shared in therapy and make their exploration less overwhelming. Furthermore, it can help equalize the inherent power dynamic in therapy when therapist and client cocreate art together.

Expressive arts therapy differs from training in the focused creative arts therapies (e.g., art therapy, dance movement therapy, music therapy, etc.) in that it takes a broad exploration of creativity across art forms, while singular art therapies delve deeply into their area of specialization. In this way, as articulated by the founders of the field, transformation is in the mindful total expression across art forms. I often think of it as piecing together a quilt. Each piece of fabric is beautiful and tells a story of its own; however, when a variety of fabrics of different hues with different stories come together in a pattern, the quilt becomes much more nuanced and striking than the individual pieces separately.

Personally, I came to the field of expressive arts therapy as a spoken word poet and dancer with a lifetime of creative experiences rooted in my culture as a cis Black American Generation X woman from South Central Los Angeles. I grew up with the southern old-school wisdom of the women in my family from Texas and Mississippi, infused with the hip-hop culture of the early 80s, 90s and beyond. I grew equally from planting gardens of collard greens and tomatoes in the backyard with my family, as I did from listening to MC Lyte, Whodini, YoYo, and NWA on the radio. My family was big and loud and expressive! Moving from making a pot of pinto beans and a pan of cornbread, to learning the latest dance step from an older cousin, to practicing lines of a play my grandmother had written for all her grandchildren to perform in church the next day were all common activities in my family. Expressive arts therapy was a natural road before I even knew of the field.

When I found the Expressive Arts Therapy (EXA) program at the California Institute of Integral Studies (CIIS), I had just started a community-based organization called Creation Cocoon for Girls, which taught girls empowerment through creative arts. The organization was designed as an after-school enrichment program held in after-school programs throughout the various communities in Oakland, CA. I worked with Black girls in East Oakland, first-generation Chinese girls in Chinatown, and first-generation Latina girls in the Fruitvale district. Everywhere I went, two things were happening: first, the girls felt seen and safe, and second, they began disclosing personal trauma histories. I knew at the time I was not equipped to appropriately respond to their narratives, so I looked for a mental health training program and happened upon the EXA program at CIIS. I realized I could take all of my experiences in the community, and my training in the arts (both formal and informal) and weave them together to create healing spaces for communities of color for which traditional therapy seemed too stiff and unfamiliar. Here began the training that changed my life and has afforded me the best career I could have ever imagined having.

Basic Qualifications Needed to Enter into the Expressive Arts Therapy Field

A bachelor's degree is one of the basic requirements for entering into a master's program focused on Expressive Arts Therapy. Typically, expressive arts therapy is a concentration of a larger umbrella program in Counseling/Clinical Psychology or Counselor Education. So, it is therefore helpful to have taken at least one or two introductory psychology or related courses. I have seen students come into the field of expressive arts therapy with a background in majors across the board from bachelor's degrees in any of the arts modalities to Human Development, Education, Social/Human Services, or Business Administration – like me.

It is also important to have a background in a few different arts modalities. Individuals who tend to be drawn to a variety of art forms are frequently excited about not having to choose to focus on one art modality over the other, and in fact, are often already cross-pollenating their artistic interests. A background in an arts modality can mean either formal or informal training. For instance, I have formally taken dance throughout my life, but learned West African dance by attending dance classes in the community. I started writing poetry on my own, but then attended one year of an MFA in Creative Writing program. Having a mixture of different experiences in different environments can provide a nice diversification of experiences.

Also having experience working directly with diverse communities is a plus. Whether you have volunteered at a senior center, worked at a suicide hotline, provided sexual health education at an LGBTQ center, or worked at a culturally diverse after-school program, any experience working directly with the community can expose you to variety of ways that people live their lives. Having an interest in social justice and attuning yourself to life experiences different than your own is helpful for expanding your perspective of the world and increasing your capacity for empathic attunement.

Finally, having what I like to call the expressive arts attitude is important. It's essentially the ability to not take yourself so seriously – a willingness to engage with cultural humility, playfulness, humor, and compassion. It's also the ability to notice the little acts of creativity all around you – to engage in your life in a creative way such that something as mundane as grocery shopping can be a vibrant, colorful, sense-ational experience.

What Is Involved in Expressive Arts Training and Education?

Typically training in expressive arts therapy is overlaid with a training in a master's degree program in counseling, psychotherapy, and/or mental health. There is also an Expressive Therapies PhD offered at Lesley University. Which type of master's level training offered is usually dictated by the state in which the training is being offered. Some states prioritize training as a Licensed Professional Counselor (LPC) or Licensed Mental Health Counselor (LMHC), others provide training in Marriage and Family Therapy (MFT). Each of these programs have a basic clinical training component in which you might take courses in: Theories of Psychotherapy, Therapeutic Clinical Skills, Human Development, Psychopathology / Psychological Assessment, Multicultural Counseling, Law & Ethics, Substance Dependence Assessment, Human Sexuality, Community Mental Health, etc. Additional training, depending on the focus of the degree, may include: Group Dynamics & Therapy, Family Dynamics, Couples Counseling, Child Therapy, Careers Counseling, Psychometric Theory & Assessment, etc.

Specific expressive arts-based training could include trainings in specific approaches, such as Intermodal Expressive Arts Therapy developed by Stephen and Ellen Levine, Person-Centered Expressive Arts Therapy developed by Natalie Rogers, Tamalpa Life-Art Process developed by Daria Halprin, Narradrama developed by Pamela Dunne, Narrative Expressive Arts developed by Shoshana Simons and Danielle Drake, etc. Expressive arts training typically includes a weaving of the five core arts modalities (visual arts, music, dance, drama, and poetry) plus other arts such as digital arts, trauma-informed arts, ritual-based arts, expressive arts in health care settings, etc.

Employment Settings for Expressive Arts Therapists

People often wonder what a career in expressive arts therapy can look like. Honestly, it takes the form of the person shaping the career. Expressive arts therapists work in a variety of settings including schools, hospitals, rehabilitation centers, senior care facilities, prisons, and community mental health agencies both government and non-profit based. Some individuals choose to work in private practice where they own their therapy businesses. Other individuals choose to use their training primarily to provide workshops to groups in the community or leadership trainings or expressive arts retreats to corporations. Some expressive arts therapists prefer to work with individuals, others prefer working with couples or families, groups or communities, or mixes of different demographics. The point here is that each expressive arts therapist often finds their own niche and has the opportunity to provide services in the way that best meets the needs of the targeted population and the temperament of the therapist.

Practicum, Internship, and Post-Graduate Hours for State Licensing and Registrations

Most states require a clinical practicum experience prior to awarding a degree in a counseling or mental health field. The practicum experience is designed to provide direct service experience providing psychotherapy/mental health services in the community supervised by a licensed professional prior to graduating from the degree program. The number of hours both direct service (hours directly providing services to individuals, couples, groups, and/or families) and total hours (hours including direct service hours, supervision hours, documentation, reporting, treatment planning, advocacy hours, etc.) vary depending on state requirements. Additionally, most states require internship/associate hours post-graduation supervised by a licensed professional prior to taking a licensing exam. Again, these required hours, both the number of hours required post-graduation and the number of supervision hours by a licensed professional, vary by state. Additionally, the accepted type of license held by the licensed professional varies by state, so these are all things to consider when making a decision regarding the expressive arts therapy training program you may want to select.

Expressive Arts Professional Registrations and Designations

Professional registrations and designations provide a level of certification for the field different from, and sometimes over and beyond, the licensing requirements of a particular state. The professional registering body for expressive arts therapists is the International Expressive Arts Therapy Association (www.ieata .org). They offer registrations as Registered Expressive Arts Therapist (REAT) and designations as Registered Expressive Arts Consultant Educator (REACE). As per the IEATA website,

> The REAT® track is designed for those who use the expressive arts in therapy. To become a REAT®, an IEATA member must meet rigorous criteria – including education, experience, demonstrated competencies, personal engagement in expressive arts therapy, and letters of reference – and agree to abide by the REAT® code of ethics.
>
> *(www.ieata.org/what-is-reat)*

For the REACE designation, IEATA states,

> The REACE® designation includes expressive arts consultants and educators who use the expressive arts in a broad range of approaches in education, organizational development, health fields, and more. The REACE® candidate may have formal training or acquired experience by applying their skills in work situations. The applicant will choose one of two application

tracks that best fits his or her education and experience. REACE applicants must thoroughly document education, work experience, expressive arts training, and personal and professional competency as an expressive arts consultant/educator and agree to abide by the REACE® code of ethics.

(https://www.ieata.org/what-is-reace)

Conclusion

Expressive arts therapy offers a flexible and creative option for individuals who are interested in pursuing an arts-based career. Having a passion for the psychological processes of people in a variety of life transitions, cultivating a strong sense of compassion for diverse communities, and curiously engaging in a variety of arts training opportunities can prepare interested individuals for a career in this field. Expressive arts therapy is a wonderful career choice and affords opportunities for lifelong growth, ever-expanding creativity, and a sense of meaning stemming from working with people as they find healing and wellness through engaging in the wide array of arts.

References

International Expressive Arts Therapy Association. (2020, December 31). What is REACE? https://www.ieata.org/what-is-reace

International Expressive Arts Therapy Association. (2020, December 31). What is REAT? https://www.ieata.org/what-is-reat

Knill, P. J., Nienhaus, B. H., & Fuchs, M. N. (2004). *Minstrels of soul: Intermodal expressive therapy.* EGS Press.

Pashler, H., McDaniel, M., Rohrer, D., & Bjork, R. (2008). Learning styles: Concepts and evidence. *Psychological Science in the Public Interest, 9*(3), 105–119.

CHAPTER 3

FINDING SUCCESS

Sally Bailey, Nancy Sondag, Lynn Chapman, Alexa Palmer, Kelly Rae Powell, and Tim Reagan

Introduction

After graduating with a degree in creative arts therapy, young creative arts therapists (CATs) are faced with finding their first job and developing their professional skills. Nancy Sondag, a drama therapist, has directed creative arts therapy programs for years and provides insight into what an employer is looking for in a potential hire. Dance/movement therapist Lynn Chapman shares what it was like to start her career in a state in which there were not many dance/movement therapists: making connections and finding part-time jobs that slowly developed into full-time employment. Kelli Rae Powell, a music therapist, explains the importance for early career CATs to find a good supervisor to guide them through their first years of practice. Alexa Palmer, also a dance/movement therapist, emphasizes the necessity of keeping your dream alive when you run into career obstacles. Finally, drama therapist Tim Reagan talks about the challenges of transitioning from working with one population of clients to a new one that you have never worked with.

DOI: 10.4324/9781003035664-3

LANDING A JOB AS A CREATIVE ARTS THERAPIST

▶ by Nancy Sondag

Nancy Sondag, LCAT, RDT-BCT, CDP develops creative arts therapy programs for persons with dementia; directs drama therapy in NYC healthcare facilities, schools, and churches; supervises and trains students and professionals; and is an adjunct professor at Kansas State University.

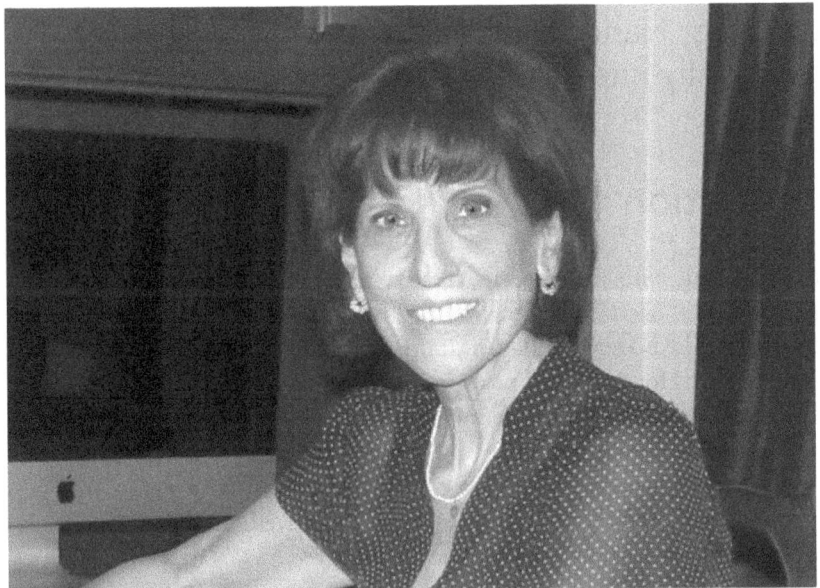

Figure 3.1 Drama Therapist Nancy Sondag.

In the twenty years that I have been a registered drama therapist, I have had the opportunity to sit on both sides of the interview desk. For fifteen of those years, I was directing programs in recreation or creative arts therapy and responsible for hiring therapists.

I have an open position now. Who am I looking for?

- Someone who really wants this job, not any job, *this* job. That means do your homework to find out if this really is the job you want. Tell me why you are suited for the job in your cover letter. When we interview, don't spend our precious interview time having me explain the job. Yes, you should definitely have questions to ask me, and those questions should reflect your knowledge of the company, its mission and vision, and the population you will be serving. You can easily research this on the internet.

- Someone on a career track. I am looking for someone who wants to grow in this profession. Even if the job I am offering is entry level, and you do not have a degree, credential, or license, I am still looking for someone who is building their career in this profession. Why are you on this career track? What compels you to this profession?

- Someone who wants to be mentored. This is a two-way street. I had some amazing mentors along the way. Not everyone in a hiring position will want to or be able to mentor you. I had a good eye for people who could mentor me and was able to win their support and, consequently, have become a good mentor myself. Believe me, there are few things as satisfying as hiring someone who is talented, has a passion for the work, and is willing to be mentored. Keep your eyes open for an opportunity where you will be mentored. If there is no one to mentor you on the job you accept, find a mentor elsewhere.

- Someone with an excellent track record. Don't waste an internship or a volunteer opportunity. If you are interning and have been trained by me, and you are reliable and a star, and a job opens up, who do you think will be the first person I interview? You!

  If a job doesn't open up where you are interviewing, one is opening up somewhere. We creative arts therapy directors all know each other. Once when I had a job opening, I got a call from a friend who was a director at another facility. He said, "I hear you have an opening. This semester, I had a stellar intern, Michelle, who is applying for that position. You would be very lucky to get her." Guess who I hired? Michelle!

  If you are long past being an intern or you're new to the profession, the same thing applies. Your track record follows you. I have worked with some talented, creative people who sabotage their career by consistently being late or calling out from work. This just doesn't work in healthcare. You have too many people following a schedule which goes all amok when you show up late.

- Someone with a great personality. Remember Michelle who got the glowing recommendation from her intern supervisor? The job opened up in June when I was flooded with recent grads applying for the job. After screening resumes and interviewing, I had four candidates who I could have hired. While the other three had good personalities, I just knew that Michelle would bring so much joy to the workplace for me, her coworkers, and our clients. She never failed me. Everyone thanked me for hiring her.

A great personality is a trait that can be acquired. Don't limit your chances by being depressed, resentful, pessimistic, or feeling entitled. Be good to yourself. Find a therapist, counselor, or support group.

Good luck! I wish you joy and success in your career. I'll end with a quote from Dr. Howard Thurman:

Don't ask what the world needs. Ask what makes you come alive and go do it.

Because what the world needs is people who have come alive.

BUILDING YOUR IDENTITY AS A CREATIVE ARTS THERAPIST

▶ by Lynn Chapman

Lynn Chapman, MA, LMHP, BC-DMT is a board-certified dance/movement therapist and licensed mental health professional who lives and works in the Boston, Massachusetts area. She focuses on incorporating the body in the process of healing from trauma and loss. She currently works with adults who experience severe and persistent mental illness.

Starting Out

As I stepped out into the world with my master's degree in dance/movement therapy (DMT), I also embarked on another change: I moved to a new state. Settling into a new professional role and building one's identity as a creative arts therapist is challenging in any context, and my move added an additional layer of difficulty to my process. Starting my career in a new state, I lacked contacts with local professionals, familiarity with local agencies, and a thorough understanding of the state's unique approach to mental health care. I was also the only dance/movement therapist, to my knowledge, in the entire state. It was daunting to imagine how I could create a path forward. During this time, dance itself became a metaphor for me as a professional pursuing, receiving, and creating opportunities to do the work I loved.

Don't Despise the Days of Small Beginnings

My first step was to leverage the resources of my graduate program. Through the director of my program, Susan Imus, I was able to set up a meeting with Sally Bailey, the director of the drama therapy program at Kansas State University. I felt anxious, unsure if I had the right questions, and desperate for leads on jobs. Then, I remembered the advice from my undergraduate DMT internship supervisor,

"When you pursue this line of work, make mountains out of molehills." I realized that I needed to notice all the "small" and "peripheral" opportunities that came my way and invest in them as much as possible, whether that meant pursuing a potentially valuable contact, engaging in volunteer work and sharing about it publicly, or considering part-time work that might lead to other opportunities. So, I went into the meeting with Sally with all of that in mind. That day, Sally offered me a couple contacts and some resources. Most importantly, Sally connected me with Helen Miller, the autism coordinator for the K-12 school system in the area.

Helen was largely unfamiliar with dance/movement therapy, but she seemed open and supportive. She offered me a very part-time job doing after-school movement activity groups with some of her students. I accepted. Of course, I wanted a full-time job with the title, "dance/movement therapist," but this was a start. I knew that the journey for each creative arts therapist is unique, and I chose to remain open about how my early days as a therapist would unfold.

This opportunity led to my next step of again accessing the network of professionals I already knew to seek supervision for my work. I immediately contacted a board-certified dance/movement therapist I knew and respected and asked her to be my supervisor. As a new registered dance/movement therapist, I wanted to accrue supervision hours to move toward my board certification. But I was also clear that, for me, I wanted a supervisor even for work that did not fully fit the criteria of clinical hours that would count toward board certification. Creative arts opportunities, volunteer work, or other types of settings that may not fully meet the criteria for certification hours can still be valuable and contribute to the development of our professional growth and networking. I wanted support in navigating that.

I also began volunteering. I met the leader of a residential program for women exiting sex-trafficking, and I proposed to lead movement and mindfulness groups with her participants. She was supportive of my proposal and open to learning more about what I had to offer. I met regularly with the women in the program, and this gave me the opportunity to hone my dance/movement therapy skills, my group facilitation skills, and my understanding of rapport building. Several years later, this volunteer work proved particularly useful when, working as a full-time clinician in a correctional facility, I was able to describe the program in a discharge planning meeting for a particular client. This client, and then several after her, ended up joining the program where I had volunteered, and I believe they found it to be very beneficial.

It is important to note here that, just as in any other pursuit in life, not every lead or contact will result in a job or volunteer opportunity. And even those that do may end up being different than we expected, or last for a shorter amount of time than we hoped. During the time that the opportunities I have discussed above were unfolding, I was also applying to other jobs in the area and getting turned down. That season of life was in some ways like an improvisational dance piece: I was unsure how the dance would unfold, where and when it would end, or who I might interact with along the way, but I was challenged to continue on, expand my creative capacity, and remain open and curious to what was to come. I believe it is critical, in this early phase especially, to not give up, but to take action and keep moving. Keep dancing!

Wait, This Is Important!

My early part-time and volunteer work helped me cultivate and hone my skills in facilitating creative arts therapy interventions, but I also needed to develop other important professional competencies, such as how to uphold the value of my services, how to ask for what I need, and how to practice and maintain self-care.

In 2014, Sally Bailey invited me to work at a summer camp as a dance/movement therapist. The Flint Hills Summer Fun Camp, an annual summer camp for school kids in the area, was working to incorporate the Hocus Focus magic program created by Kevin Spencer. The idea developed by Kevin and the Flint Hills summer camp committee was to integrate creative arts therapies and the magic components of Hocus Focus: campers would learn magic through all the arts and participate in daily groups led by four creative arts therapists, in visual art, drama, music, and dance. Creating this experience required a great deal of planning, and I benefited from participating in that process.

One day, during one planning meeting, I was surprised when I was asked what my rate was as a dance/movement therapist. I should have been prepared for this moment, but I was not. As I stalled for time to think, the music therapist next to me stated her own rate and what rate she thought would be appropriate for me. It was far more than I would have ever asked for! What I learned in that moment was twofold: I needed to be prepared for those conversations, and I needed to know the value of my professional work and express it with confidence.

It is often difficult to assess the value of one's work, especially as an artist and in a field like creative arts therapy. And this skill did not suddenly become easier right away; however, with practice, it became more doable for me. For example, three positions later, I confidently negotiated for a substantially higher salary upon hire. This was because I had the contextual information and personal experience to ask for this with confidence.

Sticking It Out

Also, in the summer of 2014, I started working part-time at the women's correctional facility as an activity therapist. I disliked the title of that position because I felt that it failed to recognize the fullness of what I could provide for my clients. Unfortunately, even many subsequent job titles that I have accepted have felt discouraging in the same way. It can feel invalidating, insulting, and disheartening to bear a job title different from what one prepared for during graduate school. I have seen others in my profession refuse to accept a position unless the job title was specifically, dance/movement therapy, but I felt that was too limiting and risky for me. Rigidly demanding a specific title may very well limit one's employment options and turn people off. There may be a way to hold onto one's professional identity, while at the same time remaining open to various titles. Yes, we as a collective ought to pursue accurate position titles, but we need to approach employment opportunities with a practical and adaptive attitude while we strive for more equitability for our work in the field.

I also found it important to consider other ways my needs could be met (beyond wages or pay) to support both my professional growth and personal wellness. Noticing and naming our needs (self-advocacy) and attending to our personal wellness (self-care) are important at any stage of one's working life. Perhaps, though, it is particularly vital during the early days of working small gigs, taking part-time jobs, and/or volunteering. Because that working context involves a patch-worked schedule and often requires mental, creative, and physical endurance, self-care may need to be a focal point of attention. There is no time better to establish a solid wellness and self-care practice for ourselves than at the beginning of our career. The work itself is deeply fulfilling, and those of us who chose the field of creative arts therapy know this well, but it is also challenging, hard, effortful work. We must find ways to remain healthy and balanced within ourselves in order to foster professional longevity. In the early days and beyond, it would behoove us to ask questions about what would be helpful to us, such as negotiating days of the week or time of day worked, employer benefits, clinical supervision, continuing education opportunities, and other of opportunities that may facilitate personal well-being and balance.

When working in the correctional facility from 2014 to 2018, I assessed what tasks were truly non-negotiables and explored what might be adapted to help me maintain my own well-being in that work setting. For example, I sometimes was able to choose how many groups to run in a quarter or how many people to include in a group. I also was occasionally able to flex my work schedule and that helped make room for both special creative arts therapy projects and my own self-care. In early 2019, when I started working at an inpatient psychiatric hospital, I chose to work Tuesday through Saturday instead of Monday through Friday, and often said, "no," when asked to do extra groups in a day. Of course, sometimes I wanted to say no, but the task needed to be done, and I was the only one able to do it. So, I did. Different work settings will have varying needs and vastly different cultures of support, but we must remember we need to both advocate for ourselves and contribute to the culture in which we want to work. We can practice remaining flexible, adaptive, collaborative and kind, while also establishing our limits, boundaries, and needs. I think this is how we both live in alignment and promote professional sustainability in the field of creative arts therapy – and the helping professions in general.

Introduce Others to the Work

In addition to self-advocacy and self-care, I found it essential to build a support network of friends, colleagues, supervisors, and administrators who either understood creative arts therapy or were truly open to learning about it. Educating others and advocating for the work may look like in-services, personal conversations with colleagues, a display of client work, or requests for structural changes to support the creative arts therapies. As a creative arts therapist, I have often needed to step up as an advocate for the profession.

While working at the correctional facility, I provided official in-service trainings. I usually used team meetings to do this and planned for it ahead of time by coordinating with my supervisor. These team meetings were multidisciplinary and had representatives from most categories of employees on site. I also participated in leading parts of annual training for staff and would briefly share about creative arts therapy whenever it could be related to the content of the training.

I engaged in regular conversations with other creative arts therapists, which helped us all generate ideas for our group and individual sessions, offered us a sense of comradery, support, and validation, and encouraged a culture of open discussion about the arts as a part of the healing process. Naturally, some of these conversations happened around or included other staff members. Having conversations about creative arts therapy in shared and public spaces was an organic way of including others in learning about it. When I participated in these conversations over time, I noticed a small shift in the understanding, acceptance, and mainstreaming of the work. A significant factor in this work for me was that I had the fortune of almost always having at least one other creative arts therapist in my workplace. Still, there are far too many workplaces with or without creative arts therapists on site that misunderstand and undervalue creative arts therapy. This requires perseverance, advocacy, and dedication on our part.

I also took opportunities to feature client work as a way to share about and promote creative arts therapy work. One particularly creative set of group participants once requested to "put on a performance." What emerged included mixed media of dance, music, and art. We practiced together, and I supported them as they decided who to invite. Several staff showed up for their performance, and while it was a wonderful therapeutic benefit to them to have the experience of people showing up for them and celebrating their work, it was also beneficial to the audience members, who learned more about the possibilities and benefits of creative arts therapy.

Access the Full Scope of Supervision

One of the obvious needs for any new professional in the field of mental health, and especially those of us in creative arts therapy, is consistent, high-quality supervision. Quality supervision gives us space to explore and deepen our clinical skills, support in navigating the early days of professional work, and time to process our relationships and interactions with coworkers, supervisors, and administrators. For me, I often felt a disconnect between the way that I viewed my work, imbued with inherent value and purpose, and the way that it seemed to be perceived by others, as if it were an appendage to "real" therapy. Dance/movement therapy is more than a nice "add-on" to talk psychotherapy: it represents my core professional identity, the primary mode through which I work, and a calling to a type of healing work. Most creative arts therapists have this unique gift and challenge. In light of this, I needed and wanted supervision that went beyond supervision for clinical interventions and helped me navigate the contexts in which I found myself working.

Accruing supervision hours as a dance/movement therapist was complicated for me and a few of my peers because we needed supervision that we could not get at our place of work. For both my board certification as a dance/movement therapist and my professional state licensing as a mental health counselor, I needed to seek a personal supervisor outside of my workplace because no one with the proper credentials was available there. This meant that I was required to expend my own personal time and money to advance professionally. This was very different than many other work settings, where clinical supervision is included as part of the work week and position (sometimes for state licensing, sometimes for credentialing as a creative arts therapist, and sometimes for both). I had to familiarize myself with the state requirements, including details, such as if an online video session would count or if the encounter had to occur in the same physical location, etc.

I mentioned already that early on, even when picking up small jobs and volunteer opportunities, I sought out a dance/movement therapy supervisor. I continued to work with this person until I completed my hours, but also worked with a different clinical supervisor for my state licensure. Unfortunately, I could not accrue clinical hours for state licensure with my dance/therapist supervisor due to my state's laws, and my in-state clinical supervisor was not a creative arts therapist. This meant even more expense and time on my part completing two tracks of supervision, though it also meant more supervision and support! Both of my supervisors offered to engage with my workplaces on my behalf, gave me support and guidance with aspects of my professional life (not just interventions and therapeutic encounters), and encouraged me to take risks that propelled me forward in my career even when I was uncertain. These qualities in a supervisor were essential for me to advance holistically as a professional creative arts therapist and clinician.

Stay in Touch With Your Artist Self

Most of us creative arts therapists found our art forms first and then discovered ways of employing art in healing work. Some of us find it second nature to remain directly connected to our art and creative process. For some of us, though, this proves to be a challenge. With each passing year of my early career, I found it increasingly difficult to be dancing regularly. I have had to fight for it and sometimes push myself toward it. I never regret it once I am there on the dance floor, because moving and dancing for the sake of moving and dancing is fulfilling and recuperative for me. I also highly value it because it infuses my work with fresh lifeblood. I believe we will all benefit, individually and collectively, both from remembering that we are artists and from being curious about how we want to remain engaged with the source and foundation of what, for so many of us, is not only our work, but our calling.

PERSPECTIVES ON SUPERVISION

▶ by Kelli Rae Powell

Kelli Rae Powell, MA, MT-BC, LCAT is a graduate of the Music Therapy master's program at New York University. She developed the first music therapy program at Blank Children's Hospital in Des Moines, Iowa and expanded music therapy services to include adult oncology inpatients at John Stoddard Cancer Center.

Nobody told me my music therapy supervision would affect my personal life so much… Nobody said that music therapy in general would send me to personal therapy in a good way!

—"Eileen," a music therapy intern

The Intern and the Intern Supervisor

Susan Feiner writes that the relationship between the music therapy intern and the intern supervisor is one of the most important and potentially transformational relationships interns will have in their career (2001). This was absolutely my experience as an intern. I trained to be a music therapist in a program that emphasizes the importance of supervision and provides multiple supervisory experiences for their students. As a music therapy intern at a cancer hospital, I had an on-site supervisor who directly supervised my clinical work and would meet with me for formal supervision one hour per week. I also had an off-site supervisor who visited me on three occasions. The off-site supervisor would shadow me for an hour or two while I visited my patients and then have a one-hour debriefing with me. She also met with my on-site supervisor separate from her meeting with me.

In addition, I had an academic internship supervisor. My class was divided into small groups of interns who were then assigned to an academic internship supervisor. These groups met weekly, and, under the guidance of our academic internship supervisor, we could share and learn from each other's internship experiences.

My Perspective as a Music Therapy Intern in Supervision

"Oh, I get it, now!" my patient (we'll call her "Janice") said to me. "You sneak the therapy into my room with the music!"

I was a music therapy intern at a cancer hospital, and I had been working with Janice for roughly three weeks. She was in her early forties, and, instead of traveling to Europe as originally planned, she lamented being stuck in a hospital room while everyone else "gets to live their life." She was an exacting person. She loved to draw little boxes by the songs on my song list that she didn't know, and when I visited her and played the song for her, she loved to mark a neat little "x" in the box to indicate it was a song she now knew. She would prepare herself for our session comfortably in her bed or in her chair. As I played songs for her, she would visibly relax. Sometimes she would smile and close her eyes as if she was really allowing herself to soak up the sounds of the acoustic guitar and my voice. She was always very appreciative at the end of the session, saying things like, "That was so relaxing!" or "Your voice is so beautiful!"

On this day, however, she didn't want a song. She was in a "bad mood." She was frustrated with family members who kept visiting her even when she directly asked them not to. She was frustrated that she wanted to plan a trip to Europe but could not. Instead of listening to music like usual, she spoke to me for roughly 45 minutes about her frustrations and irritations. She danced around the unspoken fear – the elephant in the room – that she might be dying. I listened empathetically to her. I validated her feelings. That's when she figured me out.

"Oh, I get it, now!" she said. "You're a real therapist! Only you sneak the therapy into my room with the music!"

We both laughed at her discovery, and it was an excellent opportunity for me to further expand on how music therapy can support adults in treatment for cancer.

The American Music Therapy Association (AMTA) defines music therapy as "the clinical and evidence-based use of music interventions to accomplish individualized goals within a therapeutic relationship by a credentialed professional who has completed an approved music therapy program" (American Music Therapy Association, 2006). Though it is true that the experience of making music can result in many positive effects, such as lowered heart rate or decreased perception of pain, music therapy can be more than a tool to achieve those non-musical goals. Music itself can be the goal. Music-centered music therapy is "deeply rooted in one's personal experience in music" (Aigen, 2014, p.18). The goal of music-centered work is "the achievement of experiences and expression specific and unique to music. In this view, the clinical and the musical are not separable. What is achieved through the music cannot be approached in any other way because musical experiences and expression are the goals of therapy" (Aigen, 2014, p. 20).

Janice already understood that music, in and of itself, can be therapeutic. Music in the hands of a music therapist can be a tool to achieve non-musical goals. Music can support the building of a therapeutic relationship between Janice and her music therapy intern and facilitate the music therapist intern in meeting a patient's needs in the moment. Janice would select songs with certain themes based on how she was feeling each day. When she was feeling anxious or scared, she would ask me to play "Let It Be" by the Beatles. She said that song grounded her. Janice appeared to need a modicum of control in her life, and as her music therapy intern, I could supply a scenario wherein Janice was in complete control. Through listening to and discussing songs, Janice began to trust me enough to use me as a sounding board to express her frustrations, fears, and desires.

This was work I loved but holding the space for so much pain and fear – especially with Janice who was so close to my own age at the time – took its toll. I recall losing weight at the beginning of my internship. Anxiety I was experiencing as I moved throughout the hospital made me feel nauseated. Dread I experienced the nights before I attended my internship kept me from sleeping well. One of my supervisors suggested this might be an issue with my boundaries. I was empathizing with my patients on chemotherapy and experiencing their side effects! After this was brought to my attention, my appetite returned. I learned that I can be there for my patients without taking on their suffering. This was a huge breakthrough for me as a novice therapist and a lesson that had great impact on my personal life, as well.

Earlier in my internship I had another experience that filled me with doubt in my own abilities. I was in the "shadowing" phase of internship, which meant I was following and observing my on-site supervisor as he provided music therapy services. During a session, my supervisor played guitar and sang for a young man (we'll call him "James") who was suffering with mucositis, a painful side effect of chemotherapy that can make your mouth very sore. During the music, James began to vomit. He began to moan, as well. I became dizzy and had to brace myself against the wall, afraid that I would pass out. My supervisor stood with James, silently, as the nurses made James more comfortable.

My inner monologue went something like this: What are we doing here? How are we helping? Are we in the way? Are we hurting him more? Get it together, Kelli! This is *not* about you! Do *not* pass out!

Roughly twenty minutes later, James was finally more comfortable. He fell asleep as my supervisor played him soothing music on the acoustic guitar. I calmed myself by leaning against the wall, humming along with the music. It was the end of the day, so my supervisor and I wouldn't have time to debrief. He excused me saying we would meet first thing in the morning for my weekly one-hour supervision.

I was miserable. I felt I had failed James. I worried what my supervisor thought of me. I dreaded supervision in the morning, assuming my supervisor was going to explain that he appreciated how hard I was trying, but that I just wasn't cut out to be a music therapist in a medical setting. I was fully prepared and even expecting my supervisor to suggest I find a different internship site. I couldn't have been more wrong. First off, my supervisor had no idea how upset James' session made me. He didn't know about my inner panic and struggle and assumed I was quietly observing his work. He shared with me that he had known James for some time and that he knew acoustic guitar often helped James feel relaxed. He was also situated closely enough to James be able to hear him say, "Please stay," which I hadn't heard. Most importantly, my supervisor normalized my fear. He said, "Hospitals can be so scary! Even when you've worked in one for many years." He said that I was being extremely hard on myself.

"Give yourself a break, Kelli Rae," he said. "You are not a robot. You are a person."

He underscored that fear is okay and totally natural to feel in the face of pain and suffering. He also stressed that if I let myself feel afraid without punishing myself for it, the fear would pass more quickly. Before this supervision I had never considered that the way I speak to myself in my head could be harmful or helpful.

Later that week, in my academic internship supervision group, I relayed what happened to my fellow internship students. They normalized my feelings of fear, as well. They, too, often felt afraid or had feelings of not being "good enough" at their internship sites. After my fellow students were done sharing, my academic supervisor added something that to this day echoes in my head as I move throughout the hospital where I am currently working. She looked into my eyes and said simply, "You are enough, Kelli Rae. You are more than enough."

My Perspective as a Professional Music Therapist in Supervision

Now, as a music therapy professional, I continue to depend on professional supervision to ground me in my clinical work, to keep me inspired, to continue my growth and learning, and to help me navigate the often messy and sometimes toxic professional world. My current professional supervisor is a music therapy professor at New York University and music therapy practitioner. We meet for monthly one-hour Facetime appointments. Professor Feiner also hosts a professional supervision group. A few professional music therapists join her in person in New York City, but others, including myself, join remotely from locations in the Midwest and the tristate area. This group of seven music therapy professionals meets monthly for two hours.

As a professional, I have found that supervision is still transformative. On more than one occasion I have found it profoundly life-saving! It is difficult to pioneer a field in a large medical setting where I am "the only one" who does what I do. It is common that a facility will only have one music therapist, so it can be enormously validating to have the opportunity to speak regularly with other music therapists who are often facing problems similar to mine. Suddenly, I am no longer "the only one." In this type of group supervision setting, we are "all in it together."

As one of my esteemed music therapy colleagues says during our group supervisions, "Music therapy is so hard!" It is! A music therapist in a medical setting is often holding very difficult space for our patients. Our patients are chronically ill, their lives are being disrupted, they are suffering from pain and fear, and a few of them are dying. We create strong therapeutic bonds with people of all ages who are in the midst of health crises. We enter their hospital rooms with our guitars, chimes, and meditation drums. The music we create with and for our patients is often beautiful and can sometimes be described using Maslow's term "peak experience." It is an honor to do this work – bringing beauty and humanity into the often cold and sterile world of a hospital. But even so, the work is still very, very hard.

My Perspective as a Supervisor of Music Therapy Interns

No longer a music therapy intern, I am a board-certified music therapist (MT-BC) and licensed creative arts therapist (LCAT) working in a hospital in the Midwest. I provide music therapy services for pediatric patients on the inpatient floors and in the clinics, and for adult inpatients who are undergoing treatment for cancer.

In terms of my orientation, I am a humanist. This means that I base my clinical practice on the principles of humanist psychotherapists, such as Abraham Maslow and Carl Rogers. As Carl Rogers says, "Change appears to come about through experience in a relationship… If I can provide a certain type of relationship, the other person will discover within himself the capacity to use that relationship for growth, and change and personal development will occur" (Rogers, 1961, p. 33). I attempt to provide a safe and supportive environment where each patient can feel supported and therefore be able to express their feelings and needs. As soon as possible, I want that patient to know that they are seen and heard by me. This is also true with the interns that I supervise. I do my best to see them, to meet them where they are, and to follow their lead. I am a sounding board and a facilitator for my students as they navigate the hospital and the type of clinician they want to become.

I am supervising a student, we'll call her "Eileen," and she has said this about her experience of music-centered music therapy in her supervision with me:

> [My supervisor and I began my supervision] discussing my logs for that week. In my self-assessment I had written about a session where, while I was providing soothing music at the bedside on voice and guitar, the patient's mother was on the phone. I couldn't help but hear the mom talking about a strained relationship with her siblings, and I felt countertransference about my own strained sibling relationship. When [my supervisor and I] started talking about this in [my] supervision, I began to get emotional and was unable to talk about what feelings were brought up because of how hard it is for me to talk about that relationship. [My supervisor] placed the bells in front of me at that point, and I started playing while [my supervisor] supported me on the guitar. I remember playing the bells in a slow and rhythmic way, and as I did this, I could feel myself starting to cry…. While we were playing, I was only focused on the music, and I felt like the experience was almost "out of body," as my head filled with the music. I had stopped crying by the time the music came to an

end… [My supervisor] didn't ask a lot of questions, and I didn't say a lot afterwards, but I remember feeling lighter after the music because I felt that I had let my emotions release through the crying and playing.

When we did talk, it was about countertransference and being aware of the potential feelings that can surface when working with patients. [My supervisor] encouraged me to look into personal therapy and delve into these feelings in order to be better aware and have some healing in my own personal life. (E-mail correspondence, February, 2020)

Later in our work together, my intern Eileen arrived for supervision a few minutes late. She was pacing and seemed to be wringing her hands. I motioned to the drums I had set up around the conference room where we meet each Tuesday morning for supervision. Before we played, I asked her if she was "okay."

"Yes!" she said brightly. "I'm fine!"

I invited her to play however she wanted for as long as she wanted. I told her I would listen to her, and perhaps join her if it felt appropriate. Eileen chose the chimes. She played a steady rhythm, and I joined her with what I hoped would be slow, deep, and grounding chords on the guitar. Her music, a minor melody, remained steady, slow, and rhythmic as tears began to freely fall down her face. I asked her what was happening. She shared with me that the evening before as she was listening to the students in her supervision group talk about their goal writing and planning at their internships, she became worried that she didn't do that kind of planning in her internship setting. She shared she became afraid that learning music therapy in a humanistic setting might hurt her chances of employment. I noticed she said "setting," but I am the humanist, not the hospital. Did she regret choosing me as her supervisor? I felt a small sting of apprehension. A humanistic music therapist absolutely sets care goals, short-term and long-term, for patients. Perhaps I wasn't being clear about this aspect of our work? I wondered in a flash if I was disappointing her? I took a deep breath and said to myself as I listened to her fears, "You are enough, Kelli. You are more than enough." Then I was able to return my attention fully to Eileen. I wanted to interrupt her and "fix" it. But I knew this fear was something she had been carrying, so I remained silent to allow her to express the fear and hopefully begin to let it go. I was glad she felt safe enough to share her fear with me. I listened empathetically. I could recall being her age and not knowing where I would find work or where I was going to live.

I validated her feelings. "It is really scary not to know where you will work," I said. I had already handed her a box of tissues. "Especially for someone who loves to plan!"

She smiled through her tears. She expressed that it felt like "torture" not to be able to plan for her "next steps." I made the decision that once Eileen had told me all she needed to tell me, that I was going to try and help her reframe her situation. I also planned to ask her if she wanted more time in supervision to discuss goal-making for her patients.

Eileen wisely said to me once during her supervision, "You can't pour from an empty cup." If a music therapist is the cup, supervision is the pitcher.

References

Aigen, K. (2014). Music-centered dimensions of Nordoff-Robbins music therapy. *Music Therapy Perspectives*, 32(1), 18–29.

American Music Therapy Association. (2006). Music therapy and medicine. Retrieved from http://www.musictherapy.org/assets/1/7/MT_Medicine_2006.pdf

Feiner, S. (2001). A journey through internship supervision: Roles, dynamics and phases of the supervisory relationship. In M. Forinash (Ed.). *Music therapy supervision.* (pp. 99–115). Barcelona Publishers.

Rogers, C. R. (1961). *On becoming a person.* Houghton Mifflin Company.

FROM EMBER TO FIRE: IGNITING YOUR CAREER

▶ by Alexa Palmer

Alexa Palmer, MA, BC-DMT, LCAT is a licensed creative arts therapist, board-certified-dance/movement therapist, and graduate Laban-certified movement analyst working in New York City. She is currently working in a partial hospitalization program for adults with severe and persistent mental illness, while in private practice and publishing.

Beginning: Fire Ignited

You finally felt it. The spark that ignited your passion, that captured your heartbeat, that cleared your busy mind, that made you feel like YOU. That moment when you felt complete bliss while dancing to the rhythm of the music or luxuriating in the glow after you published your first poem, that moment when you acted in your favorite play or captured your essence through artwork.

At different stages in life, we feel this embodiment of creativity. We have the ability to sense something that's, well, like magic. Our physical existence responds to our passion. The body knows what makes it feel at home. Yet, where there is magic, there is also the potential absence of it. Sometimes we go days, weeks, months without feeling it. It can be like an amorphous blip on the EKG machine of Imagination and Existence. We try to time it right so that we can strike the match and ignite the spark again.

As individuals in the creative arts, we know deeply the immense effect of using art, music, dance, spoken word, and other forms of self-expression when coping with the fluctuations of life. It becomes the thing that makes us more human while simultaneously helping us deal with the challenges we face. It can also be the refuge from our deepest pains, our private island amongst the oceanic storms.

My Path: The Candle Burns

I first started dancing when I was three years old. From then on, all I wanted was to be a dancer. Dance became my muse, my passion, and my drive. From the ages of three to 18, I studied ballet, jazz, and hip-hop at two different pre-professional ballet studios. Most days after-school I would spend at the studio taking as many classes as money would allow. When not in class, I would practice exercises and combinations at home. I would go to school, preparing for dance classes and rehearsals. Years passed as the candle burned. Sometimes it flickered and sparked, like when dust falls into flame. The candle melted, sometimes too quickly, extinguishing itself. Through dance, my emotional life was both lulled and fueled. My art form both created anxiety and soothed it in different ways. Dance promoted an intense somatic understanding of myself, while simultaneously creating a distorted vision of my physical form. But it was through the non-verbal expression and experience of dance that I began to understand my Self and to identify a career path.

When I was in high school, at the age of 16, I felt a new kind of spark. It felt more like a firework smoldering across the sky, lingering on for days at a time. I had started volunteering at a dance studio for individuals of all ages with special needs. I walked in, not knowing what to expect. There were about six adults standing in the small studio, some with autism, some in wheelchairs, some younger, some older, some verbal, some nonverbal. We danced together, weaving across the floor in different spatial patterns, at times pausing for more stationary dance moves. Promoting socialization, empathy, structure, and organization, we continued to dance. Sparks of joy, creativity, and connection spread from hand gesture to hand gesture, from eye gaze to eye gaze. We were being with each other through the dance of the nonverbal.

At the end of the class, we all stood in a circle, and that's when I felt it. Out of nowhere, the match struck a spark. We were saying goodbye to each other, arms lifted toward the sky, as community vans and parents came to pick up their loved ones. Goose bumps crawled on my flesh; tears began to cup around my eyes. This was what I wanted to do. I wanted to share the power of dance with those who were not in society's mainstream. Because Dance is for Every Body: wheelchair bound or ambulatory, autistic or not. I continued to come back for the next six years as a dance teacher's assistant.

I wanted to fuel that fire so that it could continue to burn and be passed on to others. In a society where injustice and discrimination abound, dance and the creative arts can be a key to promoting acceptance and justice. The creative arts can be a vehicle through which we create that change. It can be a refuge from trauma, from hate, or from societal limitations. It can be the medium through which we meet ourselves and the world.

***

Feeling all these ephemeral sparks, figuring out how to make a living, a career out of the arts, can be a daunting task: one that takes time, commitment, dedication, and drive. While in college, I struggled to figure out what to major in. I vowed to major in anything *but* dance, thinking that I would be more "successful" majoring in something like biology. I switched my major daily in my freshman year, ultimately choosing dance and psychology. I was accepted into the dance department after passing our "moderation exam." But I did not make it into the psychology department. The acceptance of my "moderation exam" was deferred until the next semester due to my poor understanding of statistics. I had the option of taking the exam again the next semester, or changing my major, so I enrolled in a study abroad program where I lived in Paris, France for one semester. As graduation loomed, I began to think of my next steps. I wasn't fluent enough to be a translator or interpreter, and I didn't want to be a dance teacher. I recalled that spark that was lit about six years prior.

Graduate School: Passing the Torch

With this spark in mind, I set out on a frantic Google search for anything related to dance and psychology. I found different graduate school programs specializing in dance/movement therapy. I was accepted for the fall semester, packed my bags, and moved to the Midwest to attend Columbia College Chicago.

Graduate school began, and I was very excited to learn clinical ways in which to use dance as a healing modality. Learning the history, theories, and practice of dance/movement therapy began to create a whole new level of awareness of myself and of the world. As students in the classroom, we became versed in the world of therapy. We practiced new interventions and learned new theories, while choreographing, performing, and advocating for the field outside of class. I joined a student organization that helped to provide outreach to the surrounding communities and within the institution itself.

Eventually, as graduate students, we embarked on our practicum and internships where many of us were the first dance/movement therapists on-site. I had never considered myself a pioneer, a leader, or an expert on anything before. I almost took time off before practicum because it felt too daunting. Yet, if the ballet world had taught me anything, it was to not back down from a challenge. I persevered. I continued in the program, while working on side projects, performances, my health, and next steps.

As we were choosing our practicum and internship sites, we were encouraged to explore populations and sites we might not initially feel drawn to in hopes of expanding or confirming our interests. It was at my first practicum site on an adult inpatient psychiatric unit where I took my first steps in the field of dance/movement therapy and counseling. I had little foundation from which I could draw upon as I stepped out onto this new stage. As students, we were meant to observe and become familiar with our surroundings on-site. Over the course of three to four months, we were expected to facilitate group therapy sessions on our own. While navigating the system, documentation, and this new world, I began to feel a special relationship with this site and population. This was something I would never have expected.

For my internship, I signed up to be the first dance/movement therapist on-site at an outpatient day program for adults with intellectual and developmental disabilities. Not only was I trying to create my own program of sorts, I was pioneering the work of a field in which I felt too inexperienced. While navigating the intense interpersonal dynamics amongst staff, maneuvering around organizational misconceptions and misunderstandings of the work, I felt that spark dwindle at times. *What had I gotten myself into? Where would I be in the next few years? How was I going to survive in this field? How could I contribute anything of value?*

Nonetheless, I persevered because I knew that these anxieties would keep me from the work I felt so committed to. I knew by pushing through these anxieties, I would gain insights that would enhance my skills as a clinician.

After graduation, I continued work on my dissertation, which was eventually accepted and published. In between chapters and sections, library runs and edits, I applied for jobs. During this process, I learned that dance/movements therapists could apply for and be accepted in a variety of different roles, titles, and programs. Whether as an "activity therapist," "expressive arts therapist," or "counselor," we could work in schools, prisons, hospitals, or private practice; the options felt endless. Creative thinking became an asset for how and where I would market myself and my specialties.

After working at a psychiatric hospital for just under a year, I moved back home to the East Coast. Following months of research and applications, I was finally accepted at a job as a temporary "activity therapist." Understanding the credentialing for the creative arts therapy license was the next step to tackle. I was on my way to obtaining my hours of practice and license.

There have been many moments thus far in my short five-year career where I have experienced doubt, insecurity, and confusion. But with those moments also came insight, clarity, and connection. I had to learn how to become more flexible in my thinking and more present to the moment. I practiced being embodied in mindful ways while also learning about my interpersonal relationship patterns. These skills have helped me hone my artistry as a therapist, allowing me to meet my patients where they currently are in their process of recovery or treatment.

Community: More Flames Shine more Light

Even though I had moved back home, I felt isolated as a dance/movement therapist. I didn't really know anyone in the field. I started researching different organizations and came across the state chapter of the national organization of the American Dance Therapy Association (ADTA). I applied to be on the board and was immediately welcomed into the community. I started finding other avenues and connections through self-promotion and research.

As time moved onward, I began feeling more and more at home. I continued to reach out to schools and organizations in the area in hopes of making even more connections. I began to realize just how important community really is in the success of any artist, of any human being. I made sure to remain in contact with peers from school as I began to branch out and network professionally. I slowly began to find other sparks and flames. My network began to grow with individuals who spoke the same theoretical and creative language as I did. We would commiserate over the same obstacles and would provide other perspectives and solutions.

I began attending national ADTA conferences, and over time, started to feel like I finally found my niche in the world. I presented workshops at different venues and attended events to promote the benefits of dance/movement therapy. I found ways in which to network and gather with fellow dance/movement therapists at fundraising events. Three years later, I became the president of the state chapter board.

As I mentioned, I had never thought of myself as a leader or pioneer in anything. Yet I was hired to start a creative arts therapy program for adult and geriatric inpatient psychiatric units, where I also became a supervisor of pre-licensed creative arts therapists and student interns. Since graduation, I have consistently worked on inpatient psychiatric units for individuals of all ages and diagnoses. Through the process of practicum, internship, job applications, and rejections, I became familiar with this leadership part of myself that I never thought existed or would ever exist.

Extinguished: Rekindling the Flame

In the outpatient group program where I currently work, patients receive both group and individual therapy from psychiatrists, psychologists, nurses, social workers, creative arts therapists, medical students, and interns. Many moments exist that rekindle the flame when it diminishes.

I sat with several patients in a circle of chairs. We began by sharing our personal experiences and the benefits of dance/movement therapy, exercise, and physical expression in general. We introduced ourselves, saying one word for how we felt currently, and then described this feeling in a color. Patients requested a more upbeat playlist for the music of our group. We began standing, slowly moving from side to side. As I began to mirror, embody, and pick up on the movements expressed, we continued to advance the movement forward, both verbally and non-verbally.

A theme emerged of "expanding and contracting" our movement. We made bigger and smaller movements. Stamina is typically diminished with medical conditions and medication regimens. As we all sat down, we continued moving our arms and legs in different rhythms. We changed the intensity, speed, and phrasing of the movements. Group members were encouraged to pass and change the rhythm around the circle, highlighting and celebrating individuality within the group. Consistently moving our arms and legs, I noticed my limbs started to feel fatigued. I verbally checked in with the group, asking them where they currently felt the energy of the movement in their bodies. Most agreed that they felt the energy vibrating in their arms and legs, but not much in their torso, so I invited that energy to transition to the spine, the torso, shoulders, head, and the core of the body.

As the process pressed on, I asked the group again where the energy currently resided within their body. They agreed that it landed within the heart. I asked the group members, one by one, to place their hand over their heart. With movement, I asked them to mimic the rhythm or the quality of their heartbeat. One provided a circular, rubbing rhythm, the other mimicked an expansion and contraction. They each provided a unique hand gesture that we all repeated together.

I then asked the group what it felt like to move more expansively, as we had been moving in the beginning of the group. Words like "liberated," "expansive," and "free" bounced around the room. We highlighted these movements and discussed these feelings. I asked how it felt to move in smaller, more condensed ways. Words like "safe," "core," and "protected" were used. We discussed the spectrum and space in between the two extremes and discussed ways in which this emergent theme impacted and reflected our treatment and recovery. Patients expressed that there was an "availability to us" and "a dexterity to express ourselves without prejudice." There appeared an adaptability and expressivity to the area between the two extremes, which can typically get lost when in the throes of mental illness.

What I Wish I Had Known: Leaving the Flame Unattended

Little did I know how intense the program, licensure, and process would be. I wasn't anticipating all the bureaucratic, financial, and systemic obstacles I would encounter on my way to using dance as a healing modality. Even though I wish I had better planned my time, money, and energy that would be taken up by licensure, credentialing, and financial loans, I wouldn't be happier in any other career. As I mentioned before, I knew pushing through these obstacles would allow me to pursue the work I felt so committed to. My passion and drive were larger than those obstacles. Despite all these waves of oceanic storms, I knew I was on my way to creating a private island, an oasis, that eventually would become my career.

Now What? Keeping the Flame Alive

You've felt it. The spark that ignited your passion, your creativity, your dreams. Now what? How do you transform a passion into a career, one that is fulfilling, both financially and spiritually? For dancers and other creative individuals alike, there are many avenues for professional fulfillment. Whether it be teaching, performing, choreographing, curating, fundraising, collaborating, researching, etc., the opportunities are endless.

As individuals in the creative arts, no matter the training, path, or experience, our respective modalities provide us with a skill set that allows us to turn our passion into a career and a reality. Focus, respect, commitment, and discipline were among the tenets that I learned from practicing, performing, and choreographing dance works. I was able to set goals, both physically and mentally, and learn how to deal with disappointment and accomplishment. Through countless hours spent at the ballet bar, perfecting positions, strengthening muscles, learning new steps and choreography, I built a deep understanding and relationship with myself.

From these foundations, we learn how to maneuver ourselves in relationship to other company members and dance teachers, much like in an office or work environment. We build strong relationships. Our dance teacher/boss might set unrealistic expectations, and yet we found a way to set boundaries while accomplishing this task. When boundaries are crossed or limitations set, our relationship with ourselves begins to morph and change. We learn ways of keeping the flame alight, or ways of rekindling that fire when it starts to go out. Whether we try our hand at teaching, choreographing, collaborating, or researching, the skill sets derived and learned from our passion set us up for success in whichever avenue we pursue. With our creativity, we can find ways to bring our passion, our flame, to the darkest corners of the world.

LEARNING TO WORK WITH A NEW POPULATION IN THE TIME OF COVID-19

▶ by Tim Reagan

Tim Reagan, PhD, RDT, APTT holds a doctorate in expressive therapies from Lesley University, specializing in Playback Theater with adolescents. He is the resident drama therapist at Dominion Hospital, Arlington, VA.

Starting Out

My siblings and I dabbled in all the arts as children. My mother, a gifted visual artist, musician, and writer made sure her brood of eight children were always supplied with materials to mold, manipulate, master, and enjoy. I cherished my genetic predisposition in the arts and fortified it, earning degrees in drama and performing arts management, jumping head-first into spreading the power of the arts, first, as an advocate at an arts council, and then, as an artist/administrator for a nonprofit performing arts organization with a burgeoning drama therapy program for children and adults with disabilities. That program, established by Sally Bailey, ended up having a long-lasting impact on my work as a drama therapist. I witnessed her build an accessibility program from the ground up. She was inspirational. Sally trained and mentored faculty on the social, emotional, and learning development needs of persons with disabilities. It was also Sally who let me know that the contract work I was doing on the side was indeed drama therapy. Dr. Stanley Greenspan, a clinical professor of Psychiatry, Behavioral Science, and Pediatrics at George Washington University Medical School, recruited me to work with some of his clients on a relationship-based therapy intervention for children with autism, called Floortime.

Dr. Greenspan's approach came second nature to me. I had no difficulty getting on the floor to play and interact with children. The goal was to follow the child, engage in their interests, and encourage two-way communication. These interactions made it easier to understand a child's sensory and motor profile. I was so fascinated by this process that I incorporated it into my master's thesis. Sally convinced me that I was good at this. I wasn't sure how this could be considered work, because I enjoyed it so much.

After a few years, I was getting restless at the performing arts organization for children. I needed a change of scenery and landed a position managing education programs for a regional theater in the DC area. This lateral move challenged me for a couple years, but I became disillusioned by the restrictions and responsibilities of generating income to support and underwrite main stage productions that had little to no connection to the work I was doing. I wanted to make more of a difference. I left the nonprofit arts world and transitioned to teaching and directing elementary and secondary theater for 32 years. Even while on this decades-long path, I maintained contact with Sally, who became my mentor as I pursued my registration in drama therapy through the alternative track.

Sticking it Out

While I was teaching theater at an independent school in Washington, DC, I enrolled in the intensive summer drama therapy classes at Kansas State University. From start to finish, it took close to 10 years for me to accrue the requirements for a registration in drama therapy, which I received in 2000. Not too long afterwards, I hit a life-changing stumbling block and had a stroke in my right temporal occipital lobe. Spontaneous physical and speech recovery was kind to me. However, to this day, I experience visual-spatial challenges as I navigate myself through space. I get lost easily. I have a GPS for driving and some walking. I sometimes have difficulty understanding the concept of time and still grapple with emotional lability. While in the hospital, I had asked if there was an expressive arts therapist there. There wasn't. I was disappointed. I needed an outlet for my emotions, and the creative process was the most comfortable way for me to do this. After my hospital stay, I swore that I would do something about the lack of expressive therapies in hospitals. I turned this stumbling block into a building block and pursued a doctorate in expressive therapies at Lesley University.

Finding Success

While on this journey, I carved out a niche at the Quaker school I taught at for 24 years. I had persuaded the administration to permit a few colleagues and myself to create a course on Quakerism and Playback Theatre (PT). We proposed using PT as the central method to reflect on individual stories in order to look for the good in everyone. Students learned the techniques of PT from the perspectives and roles of teller, conductor, actor, musician, audience, and researcher. By the end of this required course for all seventh graders, small cohorts within each class presented original PT performances reflecting what they had learned about important Quaker social movements, history, faith, and practice. This became my platform: PT for and with adolescents.

Playback Theatre became the driving force behind my pursuit of learning more about the expressive therapies. Lesley's low-residency program allowed me to work full-time while pursuing my degree. Fortunately, I was able to take a sabbatical from teaching to conduct research. I graduated in four years. Looking back, I'm not sure how I did it, but I'm glad I did. Despite the success I was having using drama therapy techniques in the theater classroom, I was getting restless teaching middle school children in independent and public schools. I had a desire to connect with people outside the classroom. I wanted to work in a clinical setting. I had always felt like the odd man out, utilizing drama therapy techniques solely in the classroom and occasionally with therapeutic theater groups I directed. I decided to take a step back. My work as a theater educator was challenging and rewarding, but I felt the urge to direct myself toward more clinical work in drama therapy. I retired from teaching, volunteered at a social service organization, and began my job search.

Starting Over in the Time of COVID

In January 2020, I saw an announcement for a dance/movement therapy position at a psychiatric hospital in northern Virginia, about 25 miles from home. Since I was not a dmt, but a registered drama therapist, I hesitated to apply. However, a Lesley University classmate, who was also an adjunct professor for George Washington University's art therapy program, encouraged me to submit my application. I applied for the position and gave my pitch as a drama therapist in my cover letter. I was hoping the hospital would be open to bringing in someone like me. Below is an excerpt from my cover letter:

> With more than 30 years of experience as an expressive arts therapist, educator, and artist, I have devoted my vocation to fortifying the impact the arts have on engagement and the human spirit. From an outsider's perspective, joining the team at your hospital means working alongside professionals committed to holistic, interdisciplinary, and compassionate

mental health care across life's continuum. I know that my imaginative approach to wellness, artistry, education, and scholarship, balanced with my highly effective practical management skills, would be an excellent match as an Expressive Arts Therapist.

The imagination is a universal human experience and essential for hope, healing, discovery, and learning. The multi-modal techniques of drama therapy (visual art, music, movement, and theater) tap into the creative spirit and wellness. In my practice, I am mindful of where those have come, where they are, and where they will go. I embrace curiosity and listen to what is surprising. Obstacles, disruptions, and disturbances become entry points for participants to observe, imagine, perform, analyze, trust, remember, and heal. Drama therapy promotes action, interaction, and reflection.

My application landed me an interview. I learned as much as possible about the hospital in advance of my visit. I combed through the hospital home page, scoured the internet for information and reviews, found links to videos on hospital presentations, and even drove out there to check out the neighborhood and commute time. I was interviewed by Expressive Therapies Department Supervisor Jody Wager, a dance therapist and former president of the American Dance Therapy Association.

"What luck!" I thought. I could tell Jody was a powerhouse. My online research told me that we knew some of the same people, and we were both on similar pages of the proverbial expressive arts therapy playbook. The pièce de résistance was that Jody was open to hiring a middle-aged, white, cisgendered male – something I assumed would keep me from getting to the next phase of the interview. I was assuming that my age, gender, and skin color would be a hindrance. I wouldn't be a typical hire, but I was comfortable with that. I just needed to present my best self.

After a few more steps in the interview process, I was offered the position of drama therapist in late February 2020. Then came COVID-19. My start date was postponed. Orientation was rescheduled. Although I hadn't started working, I received a safe passage letter on March 23. It was in emergency support response to the COVID-19 viral pandemic. The letter stated that I was "a mission-critical employee tasked with the provision of vital support services at hospitals and critical healthcare support locations across the nation in emergency support response." I thought, "Toto, we're not in Kansas anymore." I had never been an "essential" employee before – ever. I did fight on behalf of the arts to make it an essential subject for elementary and secondary students. This was different. I realized that being essential meant that I had to make myself available to work all hours, as well as be prepared to travel to the hospital's other sites to run groups with outpatients. I was transitioning from a job where I had summers and inclement weather days off to a position where neither snow nor rain nor heat nor gloom of night would keep me from the swift completion of my appointed rounds.

I wasn't fully onboard until late April, two months after I was offered the job. Then, because of the pandemic, I was told that hours were being monitored closely and training would be cut short. Instead of working the original 9 a.m. to 5 p.m. schedule I was offered, sessions would be adjusted. Within a week, I was conducting my own groups. By the end of the second week, I had met with all the units: children, eating disorders, adolescents, adults, partial hospitalization, intensive outpatient hospitalization, and tele-health. Jody, my supervisor, was very accommodating of my learning curve. She was kind, patient, and very supportive.

As the pandemic tightened its grip on the East Coast, there was a reduction in the hospital census patient numbers. People were staying away from this hospital and others for fear of contracting the virus. This psychiatric hospital could only accept patients testing negative for the virus. Unfortunately, test result turnaround time was slow. Already, some of the staff and current patients had tested positive for COVID-19. The adult unit had to be quarantined for two weeks. Work hours were cut. Having received a salary for all my previous jobs, I was now tethered to "the clock," collecting an hourly wage. I had to unlearn previous job systems and learn new (basic) ones. Clock in at the start of the day. Make sure to clock out for lunch, which could be no longer than 32 minutes. Jody, my supervisor, received daily reports of department employee hours. I was corrected several times on time in/out protocols and knew I had to be mindful of them. I will, however, never forget what Jody shared with me, "Tim, the good thing is that when you go through the routine of clocking in and out for the day, you know when you're at work and when you're not. Clocking out means you're not working. Go home, and don't take the work with you."

As a lifelong learner, this was a challenge. I always took work home. Perhaps that's the curse of the teaching profession. I was always reading scripts, plotting out staging, lighting, and sound cues; visualizing and formulating designs for costumes, sets, and props; and planning schedules and meetings. I placed high standards on my work while teaching and directing. I didn't want to disappoint, a burden I regularly placed on myself since entering the workforce. Now that I clock in and clock out at the start and end of each day, I feel senses of relief and release. I can be myself and not have to worry about going above and beyond the call of duty to prove my worthiness to stakeholders. Granted, as a newbie in clinical drama therapy, I continue to do plenty of research and information gathering. I find myself adapting material from drama classes I taught, therapeutic theater companies I directed, and one-on-one drama therapy sessions I conducted with children. I make adjustments to make my expressive arts experiences fit within the scope and needs of the various psychiatric units within the hospital.

As the virus progressed, members of the expressive arts therapy team were asked if they wouldn't mind being deployed to other areas of the hospital, such as screening for C-19 at the front door, being a sitter or one-on-one for a patient, or conducting psychoeducation groups with patients. Those who volunteered would receive their regular hourly pay and be eligible to receive "pandemic pay." This was a benefit the hospital offered to full-time employees who agreed to be deployed. Those who stepped up for redeployment received their regular hourly wage. For hours not worked during a typical 40-hour work week, employees would receive pandemic pay, or 70% of their hourly wage. This perk came to an end August 1. It eased the transition for my family as we had become used to reduced take-home pay. Fortunately, our daughter had graduated college, so those tuition bills were no longer a hardship.

Still becoming accustomed to living on a lower combined income, one of my sisters said it was a good opportunity for me, "Timmy, this is a great way to transition into retirement." Two of my brothers and my sister's husband recently retired. I wasn't thinking of retiring, but my sister's comment changed my perspective. I knew I had wanted to change careers, but I was worried about making ends meet. Fortunately, my wife was born with the tenth intelligence (outside of Gardner's nine multiple intelligences) which I call fiscal intelligence. She's the wise one in the family who knows how to stretch a dollar and balance a checkbook.

I appreciated being deployed at the front door, screening for the virus. It compelled me to learn about this hospital's culture. I came in contact with nurses, psych technicians, and administrators at the start and ends of their shifts. The themes I picked up on from employees were of compassion, respect, and service. Patients admitted to the hospital and accompanied by family members, ambulance workers, or law enforcement officials were greeted with messages of hope and support from intake staff.

Today, my groups focus on self-expression and spontaneity through storytelling, story listening, and role playing. I encourage patients to call upon the mind, body, voice, and imagination to strengthen skills in emotional and behavioral regulation, comprehension, and self-reflection. Instead of implementing a variety of lessons for a myriad of students in different grade levels as I used to, I now create expressive arts experiences that can be tailored to patients in the various units.

There are a number of differences between the work I did as a teacher using drama therapy techniques in the theater classroom to the work I do now as a drama therapist in a psychiatric facility. Before, I created lesson plans with clear objectives and outcomes for children in a school setting. Expectations of my work rotated around creating project-based theater experiences that led to some kind of product, whether an informal sharing in the classroom or formal production before an audience. Now, I design more fluid expressive arts experiences for populations less familiar with the process of using the mind, body, voice, and imagination as tools for healing.

I learn more information about the patients I see now than I did about the students I taught, many of whom had suffered their own traumas or mental illnesses. Everything is context. My expressive therapies colleagues and I continually learn about patient hobbies, interests, leisure activities, and occupations. We gather understanding of patient coping strategies, goals for hospitalization, and the pursuit of activities after returning home. We regularly prepare interventions and conduct assessments of patients: patient treatment, safety, and financial accountability are the top priorities.

Conclusion

When I was a teenager, one of my older brothers developed schizophrenia. He was just 20 years old. This was back in the 1970s, when not much was known about the illness. I witnessed my brother socially isolate, talk to people who weren't there, become aggressive, experience mental confusion, hallucinate, become paranoid, and have religious delusions. This was very hard on my family and me. I've carried the impact of his trauma with me. It's a part of who I am. It's no accident that the trajectory of my career path has led me to working as a drama therapist in a psychiatric hospital. In a sense I've been preparing for this work for more than 30 years. At this stage in my life, I'm unexpectedly surprised to have made a change in careers. I like to think that the gift of the arts my mother provided her children opened the door to self-expression. My brother's illness opened the door to mental illness. I'm proud to have had the ingenuity to combine these life experiences into a career of service.

CHAPTER 4

GETTING AHEAD

Sally Bailey, Tally Tripp, Philip Weglarz,
Barbara McKechnie, Ruthlee Adler, Paula
Patterson, and Jamie McCoppin

Introduction

As a career as a creative arts therapist (CAT) grows, new opportunities for other kinds of work involving creative arts therapies appear. Writing, teaching, consulting, and advocating for clients become possible as creative arts therapists feel confident in their professional skins. Chances to expand skills appear, as CATs collaborate with each other and realize how their art forms support and expand on each other. Challenges to practice are overcome through CATs' creativity and determination to continue their development.

Art therapist Tally Tripp has become an international consultant, taking art therapy abroad to train traditional counselors and therapists in other parts of the world in dealing with trauma. Teaching has been a natural next step for expressive arts therapist Philip Weglarz. Barbara McKechnie epitomizes a creative arts therapist who has been a lifelong learner, seeking training in other creative arts therapies in order to serve her clients in the most informed and ethical manner she can. Music therapist Ruthlee Adler found herself researching and writing a book, *Target on Music*, to meet other music therapists' and educators' needs for including children with learning and physical disabilities in music classes with typically developing children. Paula Patterson began her career as a dance/movement therapist but was inspired to study other arts modalities and became credentialed in them as well. Finally, Jamie McCoppin had just created

DOI: 10.4324/9781003035664-4

her own coaching and play business in New York City when COVID-19 struck and face-to-face interactions with others were shut down. With no warning, she had to transition immediately to playing with her clients on Zoom! As she adjusted and adapted her work, she found many creative uses for technology she had not imagined and discovered that she knew how to play with anyone anywhere!

EXPANDING HORIZONS: CREATIVE ARTS THERAPIES IN INTERNATIONAL CONTEXTS

▶ by Tally Tripp

Tally Tripp, ATR, LCSW is a registered, board-certified Art Therapist and licensed clinical social worker in Alexandria, VA with a private practice specializing in art therapy for the treatment of psychological trauma. Tally is an assistant professor for the George Washington University Art Therapy Program where she serves as director of the Art Therapy Clinic. Tally's international work includes conducting study abroad and service trips in sub-Saharan Africa, along with training and art therapy consultation for the Common Threads Project.

Introduction

My first art therapy client in 1978 was a six-year-old girl diagnosed with childhood schizophrenia and selective mutism. Mary (a pseudonym) had many phobias and anxieties that made it difficult for her to interact with the staff and other patients on the psychiatric ward of the children's hospital where I worked at the time. An exceedingly shy child, Mary took to me immediately because she loved making art, and I had the art supplies. It was through the process of making art that Mary found meaningful ways to express her fears and communicate her needs. Together, we devised a graphic narrative using the drawings she produced where her idiosyncratic images became a form of "symbolic speech" (to use a phrase from art therapy pioneer Margaret Naumberg, 1973). It was through these pictures that Mary was finally able to tell her story and communicate her feelings and needs, validating the unique power and potential of art therapy.

A significant benefit of art therapy is its ability to transcend language, culture, and even chronological age. Children often have an easier time expressing themselves through art than adults who may be more concerned about making a product that looks like something. Although we often use words when asking clients to describe their imagery or experiences in art therapy, we do not actually rely on verbal expression or even cognitive skills in our approach. Making art is an inherently therapeutic process. Art therapists consider the process of making artwork equally, if not more important, than the search for meaning reflected in the completed art product.

The therapeutic process of making marks on a page, pounding clay, tearing paper, applying paint, naturally engages the artist's emotional and somatic state and facilitates finding creative responses to challenges and stressors. After the paint is dry, and the piece is complete, the art therapist and client together can explore the finished product to uncover both overt (obvious) and covert (not so obvious) messages and meanings. Mary's artwork related to her memories of childhood trauma, which were at the root of her anxiety. Once she expressed that fear through her artwork, the therapists and staff could help Mary manage her need for safety and comfort.

Sometimes the artwork produced in art therapy can convey meaning that is "preverbal," suggesting the artist is not even aware of the implicit message or not willing to face the underlying meaning. An art therapist must be adept at "reading artworks," with the caveat that we must avoid interpretation without the client's input. Likewise, symbols and colors can be both cultural and personal, so we must be careful not to project our own assumptions onto the work of another.

Art therapy has the ability to communicate beyond the boundaries of language and culture, allowing us to work within a range of diverse contexts. I have taught and consulted in many international settings where art, and the feelings generated from the art-making process, was the glue that bound us together. The lessons I've learned in cross-cultural connections with art therapy is something worth sharing with art therapists and students alike.

Teaching in Ukraine

A few years ago, I taught an intensive week-long graduate course focused on Art Therapy and Trauma in Lviv, Ukraine. Since most of the participants spoke Ukrainian or Russian and a little English, I had to rely on a translator to help me conduct a series of art therapy-based experiential learnings. The focus of the course was using experiential tools to help manage traumatic stress. At the end of the third day, one of my students approached me and asked in halting English if I'd consider working with her to process a recent trauma. The creative arts approach we had practiced that day had connected emotionally with her and brought up feelings she wished to explore. She felt understood by my creative, experiential approach. It was more meaningful to her than the purely cognitive tools used by her Ukrainian psychologist. I was pleased that the experience resonated with her, but, of course, I could not accept the offer. Still, it was an experience that has stuck with me as a prime example of how creative arts therapies connect with feelings and emotions without regard to language or culture.

Winterveldt, South Africa: Bokamoso Life Centre

One of the most cherished opportunities my role as an Art Therapy professor has given me is the chance to take graduate students to study and work in South Africa. Our immersive study abroad experiences have centered around the Bokamoso Life Centre (BLC), located in a rural township about 30 miles north of the capital of Pretoria. It is also the historical capital of Apartheid. The BLC was founded by a South African doctor and his wife as a program to work with youth in response to the horrific history and outcome of the Apartheid regime. Bokamoso's mission is to provide opportunities to deal with a host of issues, including unemployment, substance abuse, HIV/AIDS, teen pregnancy, and limited educational and career opportunities. The physical compound of the center is composed of several large, bleak cinderblock structures that magically come alive each morning when the youth arrive. Some have walked the distance from many miles away to begin their morning circle with singing, dance, and prayer. It is fitting that Bokamoso translates from the native Tswana tongue to mean "Future." Bokamoso definitely lives up to its name by being a healing and empowering community resource providing hope for the future.

George Washington University's Art Therapy program began its association with BLC in 2011 through a study-abroad program in collaboration with GW Theater Professor Leslie Jacobson. To support the center, Leslie and her artistic partner, Roy Barber, created a nonprofit foundation in 2008 that funds scholarships to bring 10 – 12 BLC youth to Washington, DC, each winter (their summer) to live with US students and their families, attend classes, and conduct music, drama, and dance performances in local churches, schools, and community centers.

In exchange, GW graduate students work at BLC as part of art therapy study abroad during our summer (their winter). Students live in the township and facilitate a number of communal experiences as they work with the youth, their families, and members of the community. In 2014, we engaged a South African artist, Vusi, to lead a collaborative experience painting a large mural on a building wall that depicted daily life at Bokamoso. Other community projects have included sewing colorful prayer flags that we hung from the windows and doors, creating sculptures with scraps of fabric, beads, and wire, and making prints using cardboard, ink, and found objects. In smaller groups, we encouraged participants to explore their feelings on paper, using crayons, pencils, and paint, while focusing on topics such as family, health, and managing stress. In the afternoon there is valuable "free time" where both the Bokamoso youth and GW students spend unstructured time together. We often taught one another songs, games, and dance routines from our respective cultures. The youth proudly took us on long walks through the maze of informal housing and dirt roads throughout their township. Our work at BLC has been incredibly enriching for all of us; we have benefitted from the relationships that have developed over the years and helped to create a tight-knit community woven together by art, music, drama, and dance. For more information about the Bokamoso Youth Foundation, go to: http://bokamosoyouth.org/about/bokamoso/

Johannesburg, South Africa: Lefika La Phodiso

Another community nongovernmental organization that has been a cornerstone in the South African creative arts community is Lefika La Phodiso (which means "Rock of Healing" in the Sotho language). Located in Johannesburg's inner city, Lefika was created in response to the violence and trauma associated with Apartheid and to ameliorate the effects of poverty, crime, violence, and health issues such as HIV/AIDS. Hayley Berman, Lefika's founder and director, is a South African art therapist and social activist who envisioned Lefika's mission as 1) providing vital services and support to at-risk children and 2) training community art counselors through psychoanalytically-informed art therapy methods.

I met Hayley through a social media connection. She was eager to tell me about her work and how she uses art in her program. It is important to note that art therapy is still not an officially recognized profession in South Africa. However, Lefika had begun training lay counselors and volunteers as "community art counselors," and this model has worked well. I was invited to conduct several workshops for Lefika, focused on art therapy tools for managing trauma and stress. I have had the opportunity to return several times with my art therapy graduate students to work directly with children and their families.

In 2016, my students and I had planned on making simple, cloth "rag dolls" with the children in the after-school program. Our plan was to engage with them therapeutically, teaching them to make the dolls that would be a keepsake of a memorable day. However, at the last minute, plans changed, and the children were no longer available to participate in our activity. We had to pivot, so we quickly regrouped and invited the children's parents to engage in a similar activity and make use of the fabric, yarn, and stuffing we had brought. We invited them to make "wish" dolls that reflected hopes and wishes for their children.

Each of the adults who participated in the doll-making activity took time to lovingly create a small cloth and yarn figure, carefully considering the wish for their child that they would ultimately write on a scrap of paper and place inside the doll's body. We never imagined this change in plans would result in such a powerful and meaningful experience. The wishes and concerns the parents shared about their children ranged from hope for their health or healing from illness to wishes for their child to successfully finish school or find work. In the end, parents gifted their children with the "wish dolls," and so the day turned out to be exactly what was needed for everyone. For more information about the Lefika La Phodiso, go to: https://lefikalaphodiso.co.za/

Pretoria, South Africa: Helios Art Healing Academy

Helios Art Healing Academy is a South African arts therapy organization focused on directed, independent learning for post-bachelor's students. The academy is overseen by a psychologist, Lorette Dye, who trains arts therapy counsellors to work with clients in communities throughout the country.

I was invited to conduct a three-day workshop for a group of about 35 counseling and art therapy students in a suburban town near Pretoria. The event became even more significant when I realized that it would be the students' only opportunity to meet and connect in real time. I had prepared significant lecture material for the group that included a detailed PowerPoint slide presentation describing trauma theory followed by some well-honed case examples. Unfortunately, persistent power outages in the church where we were meeting rendered the slide show entirely useless. It was a disruptive and somewhat frustrating situation, but not an unusual experience for trainers and consultants working in the field. I had to be flexible and rely on years of teaching and knowledge to keep the students engaged and continue our learning process. We broke into small groups of about 5 – 6 students each. I invited each group to make art that would help them discuss challenging cases and concerns from their clinical work. I was able to sit in on the groups where I listened more than I spoke (a technique that is helpful with any cross-cultural work environment). Ultimately, this more personal and relaxed format led to some important connections and awareness that may not have been possible with my original teaching plan. Through the art responses and conversations, I quickly learned that many of the students in the room had been experiencing overwhelming anxiety and stress due to the great amount of trauma in the communities where they worked. Our small group discussions provided a valuable healing space for students to share their experiences and perspectives, to witness and be witnessed, see and be seen, all of which we know is at the root of healing. In the end, teaching "in the dark" was extraordinarily successful because it provided a deeper, richer experience for everyone. In our international field work, whether during a training or presentation or working with clients, flexibility and creativity are invaluable qualities of an art therapist. For more information about the Helios Art Healing Academy, go to: http://www.helios.co.za/art.htm

Experiences in East Africa: Global Alliance Therapeutic Arts Program

In January 2016 I was offered a new opportunity to work in Kenya, East Africa, as a volunteer with the Global Alliance for Africa's Therapeutic Arts Program (GAA TAP). After my first trip as a volunteer with GAA, I expressed an interest in continuing to work with the organization to bring my trauma-based art therapy lens to the program's trainings. Since then, I have made yearly trips to East Africa as a member of the leadership team, which includes Cathy Moon, an art therapist from the School of the Art Institute of Chicago (SAIC), Linda Stolz, director of programs for GAA, and a fairly consistent group of East African professional and para-professional artists and counselors that we refer to as our partners.

The GAA is committed to social justice work in East Africa. The GAA's mission is to engage with the poorest and most vulnerable populations, to find ways to help them deal with problems of extreme poverty, lack of transportation, drug abuse, domestic violence, HIV/AIDS, and lack of access to healthcare, clean water, and adequate sanitation. Art therapy in this context involves working with our partners – those providing direct services to these populations – through teaching and practicing creative arts approaches.

Each year, the TAP program brings together a volunteer group of professional creative arts therapists from across the US and other countries, who join with our East African partners for a series of trainings and skill shares lasting several weeks. Our group of international visiting therapists takes seriously the reminder to listen more and talk less, as we engage with our African partners. We learn from each other and practice culturally sensitive art therapy with tools that are appropriate for varied communities.

While most of our work with the TAP involves a training for the adult therapeutic artists, we sometimes have opportunities to work with the children as well. For example, we were invited to spend an afternoon with local school children in Bagamoyo, a coastal village on the Tanzanian coast that was once the face of East Africa's slave trade. As we had difficulty communicating verbally, it wasn't long before someone decided that taking the group to the beach would be a good way to forge connection. We set up a beach experience where we worked together in small groups to create our own worlds in the sand using found materials. There were lots of pantomiming and drama as we built, dug, and gathered materials. The children created elaborate villages using their hands to form fortresses, moats, fences and flagpoles from sand, shells, seaweed, and driftwood. Before long there were roads that bridged one community to the next, thus an expansive network was formed. The connections happened naturally as created through art, drama, and play. For more information about the Global Alliance for Africa, to go: https://www.globalallianceafrica.org/

The Democratic Republic of Congo: Common Threads Project

My work in the Democratic Republic of Congo (DRC) has been one of the most challenging and most rewarding international service experiences to date. In 2018, I was invited by Common Threads Project (CTP) founder and director Rachel Cohen to accompany her on a three-week trip to launch a CTP effort at the Panzi Foundation. Headed by 2019 Nobel Peace Prize winner and Congolese gynecologist Dr. Denis Mukwege, the Panzi Foundation provides services to women who have been victims of gender-based violence, including sexual assault, rape, and genital mutilation. The CTP creative arts approach to therapy aligns well with Dr. Mukwege's psychosocial rehabilitation model as a healing center for the women he treats.

Traveling to the DRC was in itself quite an experience. Everything about the trip was difficult from obtaining a visa to the grueling three flights across Europe and Africa, the overland transportation through Rwanda, passing through security checkpoints with armed guards and security dogs to finally arrive at our headquarters in South Kivu on the eastern border of Congo. This is not an area where many tourists would be seen, and Rachel and I were sheltered at a monastery in nearby Bukavu on the shores of Lake Kivu where we were protected behind thick concrete walls, razor wire, and a 24-hour guard on duty.

The work of CTP in the Congo is a "train the trainer" model, meaning that we provide a framework and teaching methodology for the Congolese psychologists and counselors that they will use with the groups of women they serve. After our first week of meeting together, we were happy that the group decided to take some ownership of the project and, with the assistance of one of our translators, changed the name to Kamba Moja which roughly translated from Swahili means a "singular, or common thread." We saw this as a great beginning for the group. For more information about the Common Threads Project, go to: https://commonthreadsproject.org/

Conclusion

I have found the arts in healing to be a unique and powerful resource that transcends borders of language, culture, and place. I have benefitted and learned from each travel experience, and it has enriched me in ways that are impossible to categorize. I owe such profound gratitude to my colleagues, students, and friends abroad who have taught me so much. I hope these stories illustrate the power of engaging therapeutically with the arts among people of different cultures, languages, and experiences.

Reference

Naumburg, M. (1973). *An introduction to art therapy: Studies of the "free" art expression of behavior problem children and adolescents as a means of diagnosis and therapy*. Teachers College Press.

TEACHING FUTURE THERAPISTS: LESSONS IN CHANGE AND ADAPTATION

▶ by Phil Weglarz

Phil Weglarz, MA, MFT, REAT, is associate professor of Expressive Arts Therapy (EXA) at the California Institute of Integral Studies (CIIS). He began teaching full-time after several years working as a licensed marriage and family therapist (MFT), applying expressive arts approaches in a wide-range of clinical settings, including medical hospitals, nursing homes, foster care and group homes, and community-based after-school programs. Currently, Phil is completing a doctoral degree in Transformative Studies at CIIS, which includes a narrative inquiry of birth/first and adoptive fathers' experiences of open adoption.

> To me, the classroom continues to be a place where paradise can be realized, a place of passion and possibility; a place for spirit matters, where all that we learn and all that we know leads us into greater connection, into greater understanding of life lived in community.
>
> *(hooks, 2003, p. 151)*

I love teaching expressive arts therapy. For me, there is nothing like gathering with other passionate, creative people, who are driven by a desire to integrate all their senses, feelings, and vast imaginations, to address individual and collective stories of pain, survival, problem-solving, healing, and transformation. We might jokingly compare our programs with fictional schools, like Harry Potter's Hogwarts School of Witchcraft and Wizardry or Xavier's School for Gifted Youngsters from X-men, but what I witness as a professor is indeed wonderful and exciting, revealing unique resources in each student and remarkable collective learning. As in the movies, internal and external challenges tend to draw out our strengths, like attunement, creativity, and improvisation, and highlight opportunities to grow and adapt.

Like many university faculty members in practical disciplines, I did not intend to become a professor. My primary motivation for becoming an expressive arts therapist was to work in direct, community-based mental health services. Very quickly, however, I noticed the demand for education about creative and expressive therapies, both among my multidisciplinary colleagues and with people receiving services. I have found that discussing our work often validates and encourages folk's existing, culturally-relevant wellness routines and helps them imagine additional ways to promote their own well-being outside of formal treatment. When people ask me to describe expressive arts therapy, I typically begin by inquiring about what they do to sooth themselves when stressed or hurting. As they describe these habits, like working out, listening to music, watching TV, cooking with family, prayer, journaling, etc., I highlight their sensory and aesthetic qualities, revealing that these kinds of things, which they know and use themselves, are the subjects of our field. At one hospital where I worked, other creative arts therapists and I regularly facilitated self-care workshops with CNAs, nurses, and doctors, drawing out each person's current strategies and seeing what new ideas might sustain them going forward. Also, with short-term medical patients and their families, I often found it vital to help someone make a plan for self-guided, culturally-relevant aesthetic practices that they could continue post-hospitalization, such as listening to music, telling stories, and religious rituals. Later, when I worked in child welfare, I spent a lot of time brainstorming and experimenting with parents and other caregivers to develop attachment-based, sensory-rich, and personally meaningful activities to do at home and in their communities. I also found myself leading embodied, reflexive practices for teams of foster care social workers. Like many service agencies, my employers routinely hosted graduate-level internships, which allowed me to continuously work alongside students and recent graduates in the roles of peer, mentor and supervisor.

The increasing frequency of these opportunities over my clinical career helped me see myself more clearly as an educator. Each of these encounters also further revealed the depth, breadth, and complexity of the multitude of ways people utilize cultural and aesthetic practices for personal and collective well-being, healing, integration, and change. The breadth of ideas and practices I was exposed to grew exponentially as I began working with graduate students in the university setting, who spoke from a wide range of diverse personal experiences and harbored expansive research and practical interests.

Like many authors of introductory texts, I weave threads between contemporary practices with what we know of ancient human cultures. My ambitious first syllabus for an introductory course entitled, "History and Foundations of Expressive Arts Therapy" in 2012, spanned more than three million years. In particular, I highlighted some the first archeological evidence of what anthropologist Ellen Dissanayake calls human beings' urge to 'make special' (Kaplan, 1999): a dark red, water-worn ironstone cobble found in the South African cave of Makapansgat that has an extraordinary resemblance to a human face. Apparently, this object was special enough for a distant human ancestor to collect it and carry it with them, at which point I ask students to share a story about something special they carry with them, on their body in the form of tattoos or adornments, in their pockets or bags, like key chains, or digitally, like a photo or meme in social media threads accessed on their phone. I stress that the things we call the arts today have deep roots in innate human aesthetic culture. Looking outside conventional definitions of "art" helps us to see how contemporary human beings continue to, as I say, make sense with their senses every day, especially in response to challenges. We can then begin to discuss special circumstances, like what we do in response to traumatic experience and times when we sought out someone to assist us, like a therapist, who could help us re-collect and try new practices.

In my introductory classes, I invite future therapists to join me in a critical inquiry around the open-ended question, "What is expressive arts therapy?" inclusive of the social and political forces that influence fields like the arts, medicine, social work, and spiritual practice. While we review responses to this question by prominent and emerging expressive arts therapists, I also curate a student-led survey of each of the creative arts therapies, which recognizes the dominant historical narratives of each discipline which then opens up to explorations of internal and external trends for each type of sensory-based activity. Students plumb journals, websites, social media platforms, and their own lives for unique examples of the use of various aesthetics for individual and collective healing, resilience, resistance, and transformation. I see my role as faculty as supporting each student's inquiry into the guiding question, and I profess my continued learning about these subjects and ignorance about what the future holds. As so clearly illustrated by the drastic, global changes caused by COVID-19, the future therapists I teach will be required to respond creatively and meaningfully to unforeseen situations in the years and decades of their careers ahead. My responsibility to is help future therapists feel prepared to attune, adapt, and innovate.

A pillar of my approach is to immediately empower new students as influencers of the collective learning process in the classroom. Drawing upon liberation pedagogy, I position myself as a teacher-student of the field with limitless curiosity to learn more about the creative and expressive arts therapies. I expect to learn more about the arts and healing in each class and recognize new areas of study every semester. This attitude seems to help disrupt many students' expectations about the nature of learning, especially in the university setting. Many folks report having bitter tastes in their mouths left over from punitive, patronizing, formal educational experiences, particularly for students whose learning has been previously interrupted by racism, nationalism, misogyny, ableism, homo- and transphobia, etc. My educational trauma-informed approach seeks to center each student's accumulated, culturally specific knowledge and wealth of personal and professional experience related to the arts in therapy. The primary – and most transformative – learning activity of the class has been a series of personal narratives, where each person, me included, shares a story with the whole class about the meaning of a selected art form in their lives, following the tradition of performance autoethnography or testimonio. After someone shares, everyone else crafts responsive artwork to externalize how the narrative affected them, emotionally, intellectually, and viscerally-intuitively, which we shorthand as "respond from your heart, your mind, and your gut." If welcomed by the presenter, witnesses share their aesthetic responses and any other feedback. This has become a foundational ritual for expressive arts students in their first semester. Based on feedback I receive from participants, this process allows for a profound personal and collective learning experience, contributing to relationship quality and trust, which is also demonstrative of aesthetic, attuned ways of being in relationship as future therapists. It also embodies a method of whole-person, inclusive, student-centered, and transformational learning which students can utilize in future coursework. Following each week's personal narrative and responding, we investigate how each of the five dominant creative arts therapies: music, art, dance/movement, drama, and poetry are portrayed in literature and social media. The course concludes by looking at the relatively recent codification of expressive arts therapy as a profession and degree program, as well as emerging trends, in which these future therapists can see themselves actively participating and shaping.

My current approach builds upon my humbling first formal teaching experiences, as a guest lecturer in various creative arts therapy degree programs in the years immediately following the completion of my master's. I have always been interested in teaching and find educational contexts nourish my creativity, curiosity, and extroverted personality. Luckily for me, many creative arts therapy programs offer introductions to the other modalities and multi-modal approaches, like expressive arts therapy. When I moved from San Francisco to Chicago after my master's, I reached out to creative arts therapy programs there to begin building a professional network. Many folks there were extremely welcoming and kind in facilitating introductions among creative arts therapists locally. Some contacts invited me to offer introductory workshops in the multidisciplinary approaches of expressive arts therapy. While I shared some of my favorite experiential activities from my schooling, I immediately sensed the opportunity to engage participants, who represented various diverse perspectives across the creative arts therapies, in generative dialogues about ways the artistic disciplines are interrelated and the forces, internally and externally, with which we contend, such as the politics of national psychological and counseling associations. Stepping into these sub-cultures of the creative arts therapies, I marveled, for example, at the distinctive ways dance/movement therapy students utilized their kinesthetic senses compared with ways art therapy students narrated their work. I felt like a privileged guest traveling across a multiverse of aesthetic discourses.

At one university-based workshop for art therapy students and faculty, I set up a large studio space with zones dedicated to sensory-aesthetic practices according to the five dominant creative arts therapy disciplines: visual arts, music, dance/movement, drama, and poetry. The goal was to create an immersive, interactive panaesthetic studio space for hands-on exploration and collaborative play, which was strongly influenced by my own background with installation art, improvisational theater and dance, circus arts, kinesthetic learning, and play therapy with children and their caregivers. I invited participants to develop and explore the different areas, like a living map of the senses and their related art forms, noticing their attitudes, preferences, and relationships. Then, something unexpected happened. Two small groups coalesced, each introducing novel improvisational elements which revealed new dimensions of the structure. One team used furniture to develop two large and intersecting bridges connecting nonadjacent zones. The other group crafted a boat-like vehicle in which they traveled through the space, inviting others aboard. As the facilitator, I welcomed these innovations to my design and became curious about what each group was revealing and exploring. Going beyond the mere re-connecting of artistic practices, these improvised creative actions promoted a critical dialogue about the social construction of the arts from a Western perspective and professional dynamics, like the need for more inclusive, anti-oppressive strategies in creative arts therapy education generally. I learned that some participants were leading advocates for critical pedagogies in the creative arts therapies, which strives to address inequity and oppression in service of transformation and liberation, including interrogating white European ethnocentrism in art therapy (Talwar, Iyer, & Doby-Copeland, 2004). While I had been invited to lead this event, the participants educated me and promoted my approaching all future teaching with humility, curiosity, and mutuality, and their work has had a strong, enduring influence on my teaching. In particular, this workshop dispelled my preoccupation with internal squabbles among the creative arts therapies and encouraged widening my lens to include the influence of larger social movements and intersecting disciplines, like medicine, psychology, sociology, and law.

The dynamic forces of multicultural and social justice counseling help define these intersections. As a master's student in 2002 – 2005, multicultural counseling education focused upon a competence model, based on therapists' knowledge, awareness, and skills regarding cultural preferences and practices of categorical groups, typically organized around race/ethnicity. When I started teaching in 2012, the use of intersectional identity frameworks, like Pamela Hays' (2016) ADDRESSING or Afuape's (2011) social GRAACCCEESS models, challenged the stereotyping tendency of the competence approach and promoted cultural humility, which highlights aspects of cultural identity that are most salient to the person and their context. Teaching offers an invaluable opportunity to work across generations. The first students I taught came to graduate school with a strong sense of self-determination and self-advocacy and high expectations for culturally-responsive teaching. They offered me generous feedback about how my presence in the classroom and the ways my positionality might be influencing my teaching and course design. At that time, the core faculty also integrated the learning goals of multicultural counseling throughout the entire expressive arts curriculum and instituted the practice of orienting new students with an immersive "Beloved Community" retreat, which invoked a quote from Dr. Martin Luther King, Jr.'s 1966 speech, "Nonviolence: The Only Road to Freedom":

> Our goal is to create a beloved community, and this will require a qualitative change in our souls, as well as a quantitative change in our lives.

These retreats include an interactive performance of faculty narratives, which demonstrate several methods of culturally-responsive meaning-making through the arts, transparency, presence, and self-awareness. Building off hooks' (2013) assertion that "without a decolonizing mentality, smart students from disenfranchised backgrounds often find it difficult to succeed in the educational institutions of dominator culture" (p. 26), my colleagues and I believe creative, anti-oppressive approaches to expressive arts education are essential for meeting the needs of increasingly diverse student-artist-practitioners and the people and communities with whom they work. For several years, we have been developing teaching practices, grounded in a liberatory, critical race feminist paradigm. Personal-cultural narratives are brief (approx. 5 minutes) individual performances, influenced by the traditions of narradrama (Dunne, 2006) and autoethnographic performance (Sajnani, 2013), that allow students to witness each faculty's process of meaning-making as individuals embedded within families, work, communities, and societies. Sajnani (Sajnani, Marxen, & Zarate, 2017) further elucidates how the performance of personal and social stories can organize responses to current events, offer performers and witnesses therapeutic benefits, and help interrupt dominant narratives. Our performances are inherently multimodal, utilizing a range of expressive arts, such as voice, text, movement, props, visuals, recordings, and/or audience interaction. Catharsis is common, as performer-faculty make sense of their own lived experience and student-witnesses realize that their emotional presence and embodied empathy is welcomed into the classroom.

Each year, my faculty team discusses prominent themes and approaches which give each person opportunities to explore their unique intersectional identity as it relates to the theme. For example, we worked with a modified version of George Ella Lyons' "I am from" poem to evoke our culturally-specific experiences of education. Mine begins,

> I am from salt dough, trapper keepers & gym shoes,
> from card catalogs, overhead projectors, film cameras, & computer labs,
> from iPhones, & Google docs & the Canvas LMS.
> I'm from Eugene Field Elementary, Carl Sandburg Junior High,
> CU-Boulder & the California Institute of Integral Studies.
> I'm from the City of Big Shoulders, The Mile High City, & the City by the Bay.

Other narratives have explored faculty members' completing their doctoral dissertation, aging and sexuality, spiritual development, childhood and parenthood, the experience of ability/disability, and mourning lost family members. In my most revealing, tender performance, I sang excerpts of five pop songs while narrating how my partner and I struggled with infertility and ultimately became parents through adoption. Crafting and offering these as part of new student orientation dramatically illustrates our collective commitment to ongoing personal work and bringing our whole selves into our teaching.

In March 2020, COVID-19-related school closures affected over a billion students of all ages around the world, including graduate students of creative and expressive arts therapies. Graduate students in practicum rapidly adapted their work to telehealth. Creative and expressive arts therapy students continued their coursework online while attending to the changing needs of work, family, and their communities. Fortunately, many of these graduate programs had already adapted degrees to hybridized learning, which utilizes short-term intensive in-person, collective learning lasting a few days to several weeks, combined with a variety of distance learning strategies. The program where I teach began to offer a hybrid degree option in Fall 2017. When universities began to close campuses for COVID-19, the first cohort of hybrid students were completing their final courses and preparing for graduation. When our campus closed, faculty applied what we had learned teaching the hybrid program and, like all of society, experimented with creative ways to maintain relationships in each learning community.

Even before the COVID-19 pandemic, many people I spoke with had trouble imagining how the practices utilized by creative arts therapists can be learned or performed at a distance, such as through video or online forums. Prior literature in the field relating to digital methods has focused on how therapists could take advantage of new media, like digital photography or iPad drawing tools, in their face-to-face sessions, rather than discuss opportunities and challenges for telehealth. Faculty and therapists accustomed to in-person encounters could no longer share their art materials, instruments, and props. Faculty and therapists who are used to actively participating in embodied play, dance/movement, and drama processes alongside students and clients adapted to working across virtual spaces without direct contact. How might we translate the embodied presence and affective resonance that is so integral to our work? Working across distances online, expressive arts, music-making, and writing processes rely upon the resources students or clients have on hand, often in their home.

While COVID-19 has required technological changes to everyday social life and education, this pandemic also highlights disparities in health, education, economic, and public safety caused by white supremacy, misogyny, capitalism, and other systemic factors. Creative and expressive arts therapy faculty have responded by highlighting and re-investing in anti-racist efforts within their programs and promoting involvement with community-based actions.

Amid the ongoing global pandemic, political strife, and devastating natural disasters, like the wildfires in California, I am more convinced than ever of the crucial need to promote attunement, creativity, and improvisation, and continue to prepare future therapists to adapt to whatever lies ahead.

References

Afuape, T. (2011). *Power, resistance and liberation in therapy with survivors of trauma: To have our hearts broken*. Routledge.

Dunne, P. (2006). *The narrative therapist & the arts*. Drama Therapy Institute of LA.

Hays, P. A. (2016). *Addressing cultural complexities in practice: Assessment, diagnosis and therapy.* APA Press.

hooks, b. (2003). *Teaching community: A pedagogy of hope.* Routledge.

hooks, b. (2013). *Teaching critical thinking.* Routledge.

Kaplan, F. (2000). *Art, Science and Art Therapy.* Jessica Kingsley Publishers.

Sajnani, N. (2013). The body politic: The relevance of an intersectional framework for therapeutic performance research in drama therapy. *The Arts in Psychotherapy, 40*(4), 382–385.

Sajnani, N., Marxen, E., & Zarate, R. (2017). Critical perspectives in the arts therapies: Response/ability across a continuum of practice. *The Arts in Psychotherapy, 54,* 28–37.

Talwar, S., Iyer, J., & Doby-Copeland, C. (2004). The invisible veil: Changing paradigms in the art therapy profession. *Art Therapy, 21*(1), 44–48. doi:10.1080/07421656.2004.10129325

WHEREVER YOU GO – THERE YOU ARE!

▶ by Barbara McKechnie

Barbara McKechnie, MA, LPC, LCAT, RDT–BCT, TEP is a drama therapist and psychodramatist who has worked with children, adolescents, and adults in both inpatient and partial hospital settings. She is past president of NADTA and NJACC and is a faculty member at Montclair State University in NJ. She currently works as a consultant, psychodrama trainer, and in private practice in NJ.

Beginnings

My drama and theater experience began as a 5-year-old at Rose Marie Floyd's School of Dance in Royal Oak, Michigan, where each spring I was part of a corps of ballerinas and tappers performing for proud parents. I wasn't "born in a trunk," as the Judy Garland song goes, but I did have a mother who loved theater and the arts. She took her children to see all the MGM musicals, enrolled her daughters in dance classes and, when finances allowed, took us to the ballet. In high school I performed in school plays and started a folk music group with five other friends.

I entered college as a theater major. It was a tumultuous time, full of unrest and change, and I soon left my midwestern campus and headed for NYC. I was able to stay with my sister, who was already working in the theater.

I had started psychotherapy soon after I arrived in NY, and I also began to explore other ways of healing and expanding my consciousness. I studied Tai Chi for several years with Wolfe Lowenthal and went regularly to the Integral Yoga Center in Greenwich Village. This was the 1970s, of course. I tried bio-energetic body work, Primal Scream therapy, psychic and esoteric group therapy. I was even in a Marxist Feminist Analytic therapy group. All of it was interesting, if not helpful.

Because I had left school before graduating, I decided to finish my BA at Hunter College. I took film classes but found myself more interested in acting than in technical aspects of film-making. I left school once again to train with several well-known acting teachers. I was somewhat shy and afraid of my own depth of feeling, but I loved the self-exploration, the interplay between actors, and the collaboration aspects of the work. I found myself changing, deepening with more awareness of my own experience and that of others. As I became more engaged in acting classes, it began to seem like a kind of therapy to me. Exploring a character or a scene in a class seemed to bring me closer to myself. I felt more present or even more myself when playing a role in a fictional story.

However, I never got comfortable with auditioning. Almost every job that I got was through somebody that I worked with before or who had seen my work. In spite of my reluctance to audition, I was able to get my Screen Actors Guild (SAG) card and become Equity eligible. At this point, I decided to finish what I thought would be the last year of my BA. My rationale was that this would help me feel more confident and make auditioning easier. Through a program with CUNY (City University of New York) I was able to create my major, *Theatre and Creative Drama*, using Hunter College as my "home school." Professor Patricia Sternberg, RDT-BCT, became my mentor. Pat, as I came to call her, created the most welcoming environment! It was wonderful, serious play. Through her, I was exposed to drama therapy, psychodrama, creative drama, and children's theater. I also found myself feeling more interested in and excited about theater in general.

The last year at Hunter, Pat was cochair for the annual conference of the drama therapy organization, then called the National Association of Drama Therapy (NADT). I volunteered to help and was able to sit in on several workshops. I was blown away by some of the work and saw the impact that drama therapy could have on individuals and communities.

In one presentation, Naida Weisberg, RDT-BCT, and Rose Pavlov, RDT, presented the inter-generational theater project that they had done in Providence, RI. Naida and Rose worked with members of a community of people who had emigrated from a Latin American country. Elders in the community seemed estranged from the younger members. Many of the younger generation seemed more familiar and interested in popular culture in the United States. Some of these teens no longer spoke Spanish.

In developing the play to be presented, Naida and Rose had the adolescents interview the elders, asking about their lives when they were younger, about their immigration to the United States, and about their continued experience here. Naida and Rose then created a performance based on the stories. During this process, the elders began to form relationships with the younger people, and the younger people seemed to develop a greater appreciation of their heritage. The forging of these connections and community-building seemed so much more meaningful than the little bit of theater work I had done. Later I had the opportunity to meet and form a friendship with Naida, who continues to inspire me.

I also saw a presentation by Ellen Williams, RDT. She showed a video of her work with two different groups of women: one a group in prison, and the other a group in a safe house that sheltered women and children from domestic violence. While both videos were inspiring, I was particularly moved by the one showing a woman in the safe house role-playing and, over a period of time, becoming more confident and assertive. The transformation of this woman was remarkable. Again, I was awed by the healing power of the work. I contacted NYU immediately after the conference to apply for admission to the Drama Therapy program.

Graduate School

During one of my first classes at NYU, I met my cohort: the people who I would become nearly fused with for two years. It was an amazing process. Robert Landy, director of the program and our mentor, told us that we were pioneers in the field. The thought was both exciting and frightening.

I was the oldest person in my class, starting the program a month after my 45th birthday. Initially, I felt very self-conscious about my age, but that lessened in time as the work intensified. Although students were encouraged to see a therapist, many students chose not to. This has always seemed contradictory to me. While I had already had years of therapy, I did not have experience, discounting the classroom, with a drama therapist. I did a series of sessions with Le Clanche du Rand, RDT, who had come highly recommended.

In the past, much of my therapy had been about loss. While it was freeing, and there was greater peace in the acceptance of life as it was, the process was painful, and, at times, I experienced much resistance. The contrast with my drama therapy sessions was stark. I had fun and looked forward to them. I felt the strength of my imagination and of being creative. I was still in psychoanalytic therapy during this time but soon terminated and chose to work with another creative arts therapist. This was particularly helpful as I navigated the internships of my second year of graduate school. My supervisor was Dr. Fran Levy, who was both a social worker, dance/movement therapist, and had training in psychodrama. This supervision was invaluable in forming my professional identity and in beginning to address the challenges of working in systems that were often under-staffed, under-resourced, and often dysfunctional.

I learned so much about group therapy being part of my drama therapy cohort. We spent the two years forming, storming, norming, and then, literally, performing (Gibbard, Hartman, & Mann, 1974). For a thesis project, 10 out of the 11 students in the program chose to do a group thesis performance. The process was an amazing experience, tinged with beauty, hurt, struggle, and strength. It allowed me, and, I assume, others to individuate from the group and embark on our separate journeys. I have remained connected to many in this group and feel a deep bond with and appreciation for all of these remarkable people.

During my first year in graduate school, I had the opportunity to do fieldwork with *Elders Share the Arts* and assist on another intergenerational drama with seniors at a center in Flushing, NY and children from a local middle school. The children involved were primarily from countries and cultures that have strong family connections. However, many were without extended families in this country, and many were in single-parent homes.

One of the stories told by an elder for the center was her escape from Hitler's Germany just before the war. Most of the children had no awareness of this time in history. Another story told was about challenges faced as a scout leader on a camping trip. The performance took place in the senior center with the children being showered with attention and applause by the center's audience members. The elders involved felt witnessed and seemed enlivened by the work with the students. Later, I heard that a couple of the elders began to volunteer at the middle school to help the children with reading and studies, sort of becoming honorary grandparents.

Finding My First Job

At the time of graduation, I had been commuting into NYC for several years and wanted to work closer to home. I didn't see any job listings, so I did a little research and found out who was in charge of Human Resources in the two local hospitals. A friend also gave me some information about a partial hospital that was an extension of one of the two hospitals that had an art therapist as director and a dance/movement therapist as assistant director. I longed to work with other creative arts therapists, so I wrote a letter expressing my interest and describing what drama therapy could contribute to what I thought must already be an incredible program. I got the job!

It was an exciting place to work, in spite of all the challenges. I was hired at the hospital on a bachelor's degree line and contracted to receive a pay increase to be on a master's level line as soon as I finished my thesis and graduated. Later, I found out if I hadn't done this at the time of being hired, I may have been stuck at a bachelor's level line and with lower pay, pending approval from those higher up in the chain of command.

Continuing Education

In addition to supervision with Fran Levy, I joined a psychodrama training group with Jacquie Siroka at what was more recently called the Sociometric Institute. I was amazed at the power of psychodrama, and Jacquie would become not only a mentor but also my second trainer as I worked toward my Certified Practitioner (CP) and then Trainer-Educator-Practitioner (TEP) in psychodrama. J.L. Moreno, founder of psychodrama, wrote about "The Double," defining it as the first stage of the psychodramatic theory of development (Moreno & Florence, 1964). Moreno called it the *Matrix of Identity*. In my training, I experienced being doubled in a way that I hadn't in my family of origin, my friend groups growing up, or even the created family of my drama therapy cohort. Because I had grown up with a depressed and distracted mother, being doubled by Jacquie and group members allowed me to feel seen, understood, and valued. It was life-changing. Psychodrama became even more interesting to me when I saw the brilliance of translating the developmental stages to techniques in psychodrama (the double, the mirror, the auxiliary ego, and role reversal). I had not planned to work toward further certification; I just found it healing, and I was learning new skills that were helpful in my work with patients who were dually diagnosed (mental illness and substance abuse). I also joined a small group of drama therapists who began training with David Read Johnson, RDT-BCT, in Developmental Transformations (DvT). While I valued it and joined other DvT groups, I was already very involved in psychodrama and didn't have time for both.

Something I feel was important for professional development, best practices, and even the therapist's emotional well-being is having supervision, especially during the earlier years in the field. Too many of us only complete the amount required for the RDT. I was part of a 10-year supervision group with Darby

Moore that met every three weeks. This group of DTs was so empowering and validating. It again fostered community and lasting connections.

While working with dually diagnosed clients, I found that probably 80% or more had experienced childhood trauma that was unaddressed. In addition, the life of the addict is often filled with trauma. At this same time, I heard of a new Certificate Program at NYU in its second year. I had already started taking some classes at my local college required for substance abuse counselors. I had no intention of becoming a CASAC but felt it unethical to work with addictions without more knowledge. I felt the same way about working with clients with such severe histories of trauma. Coincidentally, this was the year before the terror attacks on 9/11/2001. This not only helped me to work more effectively and safely but I also learned about vicarious trauma, a risk many of us face working in the helping professions.

After many years, I took a new job working with children and adolescents in an inpatient setting. I had done some after-school programs with children, but I felt unprepared for this work, so I sought additional training at NYU. NYU's drama therapy program offered tuition-free classes for hosting and supervising drama therapy interns. Because my new work location was in Greenwich Village, NYC, close to NYU, it was a popular internship choice for students. So, with my credits, I took classes that I hoped would help, such as Drama Therapy with Children, which was taught by Anna-Marie Webber, RDT-BCT. I also took classes in educational theater with Nan Smither in the Educational Theatre Department.

Credentialing

All these classes were helpful in terms of increasing knowledge and skills, but there was an added benefit of increasing my graduate credits so that I could meet the requirements for a brief period of "expedition" (what was then called "grand-parenting") to become a Licensed Professional Counselor (LPC) in NJ, where I was living. This was especially significant later, when I became a founding member of the New Jersey Task Force for Licensure of Drama Therapists and Dance/Movement Therapists (See Chapter Five for more on the work of the Task Force for New Jersey creative arts therapists). Although many of us on the task force had shown the equivalent in education and qualification to become LPCs, there was no longer an opportunity to be expedited in NJ for new creative arts therapists. It was time to change this.

Giving Back to Your Community

I began serving as the Eastern Representative on the NADT Board of Directors and served for 2 terms (4 years) in that role before becoming president-elect and then president of NADT (now the North American Association for Drama Therapy, NADTA). This gave me an opportunity to meet and work with others on the board and to form many new and lasting friendships. While there are too many board members to mention individually, I would like to acknowledge how much I learned from Alice Forrester, RDT-BCT, Sally Bailey, RDT-BCT, and Sherry Diamond, RDT, each of whom served as president during my first six years on the board.

Based on my experience with the NADTA, I can wholeheartedly recommend that you find the level of commitment you are willing and able to make to your professional organizations, whether it is through filling out surveys, volunteering for a short-term task group, helping out at a conference, or running for a board position. Doing so is not only an investment in your professional creative arts therapy organization and in growing the larger field of creative arts therapy, but it is an investment in yourself and your career.

In 2005 my friend and colleague Ann Smith, RDT-BCT, recommended me to Dr. Louise Montello, director of the Creative Arts and Healing program at The New School, to replace Ann as an adjunct instructor when Ann went into a doctoral program in clinical psychology. I remained there until the program closed in 2017. While every job I have had has seemed important and has added meaning to my work and career, The New School will always have a special place in my heart. Classes were considered undergraduate level, but they had a very different composition than most undergraduate classes. In addition to having many international students, they often had a wide age range and included returning adults, many who had a great love for or much experience in the arts. Many of the students in the Creative Arts and Healing program went on to MA programs for creative arts therapies.

Conclusion

I am "semi-retired" at this time, working part-time in a group practice as an LPC, using drama therapy and psychodrama. I will soon be licensed as a drama therapist in New Jersey. I co-led a training group with a music therapy colleague, Amy Clarkson, in which we integrate drama and music therapy with psychodrama.

Last year, I was invited to teach Montclair State University's first drama therapy class. This seemed significant since licensure for drama and dance/movement therapists was in process. In spite of the impact that the pandemic and economy is having on the university, they invited me to teach a second year this spring. There was even mention of adding a course in drama therapy at the graduate level.

In reflecting on this journey, the most important insight I might share is that it is never too late to start something that awakens you. Knowledge is transferable. This work keeps you young, as I witnessed with my friend Naida Weisberg. Building connections with others may take you to the next possibility. The world is full of opportunity.

References

Dayton T. (2005). *The living stage: A step-by-step guide to psychodrama, sociometry and group therapy*. Health Communications.

Gibbard, G. S., Hartman, J. J., & Mann, R. R. (Eds.). (1974). Group process and development. In *Analysis of groups; Contributions to theory, research, and practice*. Jossey-Bass, Inc. Publishers.

Moreno, J. L., & Florence, B. (1964). Spontaneity theory of child development. In J. L. Moreno (Ed.). *Psychodrama: Volume I*. (pp. 47–84). Beacon House, Inc.

WRITING A BOOK TO OPEN DOORS FOR OTHERS

▶ An Interview With Ruthlee Adler

Ruthlee Figlure Adler, MT-BC, is a music therapist and consultant in Bethesda, MD with over 60 years of experience working with children and adults with varying abilities. She created and maintained the music therapy program at Ivymount School in Rockville, MD, while also working with clients at the National Institutes of Health and in her private music therapy practice. She is the author of numerous music therapy publications, including *Target on Music: Activities to Enhance Learning through Music*. Ruthlee has served on the Board

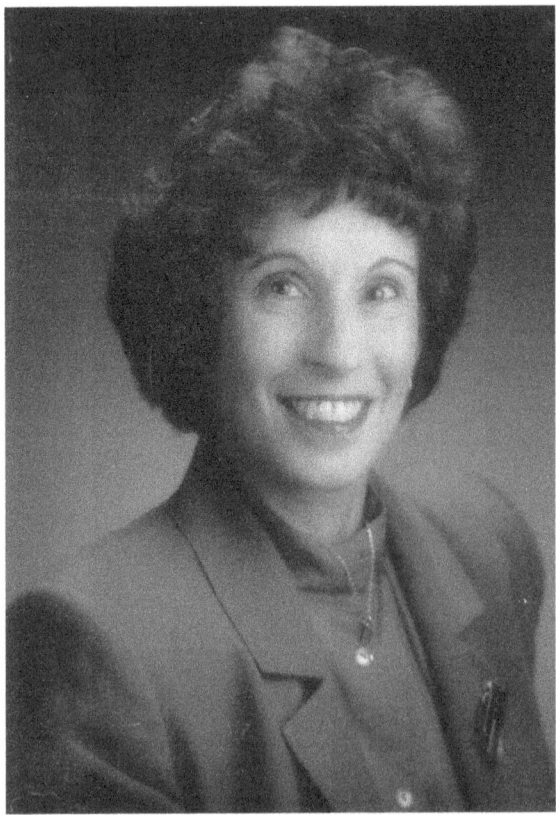

Figure 4.1 Music therapist Ruthlee Figlure Adler.

of Directors for the American Music Therapy Association (AMTA), as well as on its Assembly of Delegates, chairing committees and presenting at conferences regionally, nationally, and internationally. She is the recipient of the Midatlantic Region and AMTA Service Awards, as well as the AMTA Lifetime Achievement Award. Currently, she is semi-retired but continues her private practice; serves as a consultant to universities, clinics, and schools; and remains an active volunteer.

How did you get involved in music therapy?

I grew up in Missouri and always loved music: singing along to favorite songs, radio commercials, using scarves to dance around the house to recordings, and "picking out" melodies on various instruments. When I was five years old, I began taking piano lessons, and my parents, sensing my enthusiasm, bought me a piano. By the time I was ready to attend college, I knew I wanted to have a career in music. However, I have a cousin who was a concert pianist and from watching her, I realized that I didn't want to be married to a piece of furniture [the piano]; that kind of dedication is what it would require if I were to pursue a career as a concert musician.

I loved working with people and was interested in psychology. I'd been sharing music with others since I was twelve, so music therapy made sense for me. Indiana University in Bloomington, where I chose to attend college, offered many music degrees but not music therapy. Four other music majors and I approached the music school dean with our desire to pursue a degree in music therapy; his response, "OK, but you have to find out what courses are required and find teaching faculty who agree to come to IU." So, we did! With his help and approval from the board of trustees of the Music School, within two years, we became the first graduates in Music Therapy from Indiana University's School of Music.

Back home in Missouri, one summer I took a correspondence course in abnormal psychology, while also doing a music therapy practicum at a state mental hospital. Two little ladies, identical twins, who had given piano lessons prior to hospitalization, were among the residents. They immediately presented me with all the music literature, books, and sheet music they had saved from their studio. The man in charge of the unit called his program "Radio Therapy" because they broadcast a live thirty-minute weekly music program from the hospital on a local radio station. It was such a wonderful experience, as I was studying abnormal psychology at the same time I was sharing music with a living class in abnormal psychology.

Upon finishing my coursework at IU, I was required to complete a six-month clinical internship of 1,100 hours before I could receive my degree. I chose Essex County Overbrook Hospital in Cedar Grove, New Jersey because I wanted to go east. My future husband was working in publishing in New York City. I lived in the hospital's student nursing unit and on free weekends I would often spend time with my cousin, the concert pianist, in Greenwich Village. It was a magical time. I finished my internship, I spent quality time with my fiancé, Larry Adler, and I was able to experience all the excitement of New York City. I graduated with a bachelor of science degree in Music Therapy and almost a BA in Psychology.

What happened after you graduated?

Larry and I were married. He had several different jobs in publishing before accepting a position with Golden Books in New York City. We lived in New Jersey and our three children were born there. During those years I was able to work part-time as a music therapist in several different private schools. The highlight of their spring semester was an original musical combining the students from both programs. I fondly remember carrying instruments (including a conga drum on my shoulder), from a parking space on the street a few blocks from the NYC branch and looking back to see a group of children smiling and following me, a la Pied Piper!

Several years later, Larry became the publisher of the Washingtonian Magazine, and we needed to move to the Washington, DC area. None of us wanted to move, except Larry, but we did. It turned out to be an excellent decision for us all.

After the move, I spent most of my time being a full-time mom. My eldest daughter was taking art classes from a local artist named Jane Mason. Two brothers, with special needs, joined a younger class in Jane's studio, and my daughter mentioned that I was a music therapist. Jane called me and said, "Art is not the medium for these students, maybe you could reach them through music." They became my first two private clients – the beginning of my private music therapy practice in Maryland.

During that time, I also studied group piano teaching, following the Robert Pace Piano Method, which allowed me to add improvisation skills to my repertoire. I also took courses in Orff-Schulwerk and Dalcroze Eurythmics.

When did you start working for Ivymount School?

The children and I were at a local swim club where I met a speech therapist who worked at Christ Church Child Center, (CCCC), the original name for Ivymount School. In those days, the school was designed for children aged 6 – 12 (now they teach children and youth ages 4 – 21), and the program was designated for "children with learning disabilities and multiple needs." This was before anyone talked about autism.

In the beginning, I offered an after-school music program, paid for by the enrolled children's parents. CCCC, at that time, was located in a number of different churches scattered throughout the metropolitan area, so I traveled from classroom to classroom (in the individual locations). My car was my office. After a year, these parents began requesting that more music be included in the school curriculum.

Shari Gelman, the school's founder and director, invited me to attend a fall staff meeting. She said that I could speak about music therapy for 15 minutes, so I came and gave my little spiel. Later she called me and said, "I don't know how we are going to do this, but everyone wants music therapy."

Tell me the story of how your book *Target on Music* was created

The CCCC parents and staff wanted more music. I was only working part-time. Education requirements for teaching special populations were being updated with the passage of Public Law 94-142: The Education for All Handicapped Children Act of 1975.

Written and monitored goals and objectives were specified for each curriculum subject area, and each student was required to have an Individual Education Plan (IEP).

In those days, Very Special Arts was called the National Committee – Arts for the Handicapped. They offered grants for arts projects, so I suggested CCCC submit a grant application. Of course, that meant I would have to do the writing. I had never written a grant in my life, but I was inspired to accept the challenge. I believed what would be useful was a curriculum that helped to integrate children with and without disabilities through music. While researching for the grant, I was able to find only one other music publication that could possibly be adapted to address the necessary requirements for compliance with Public Law 94-142. I was totally surprised when CCCC was chosen as one of the final 1981 ten Special Projects. Our grant was titled, "Music Therapy for Handicapped Children." From that evolved the book *Target on Music*.

Therefore, for *Target on Music* to become a reality, I knew that it would need to be integrated with curriculum goals/objectives so that music would ultimately be included on the IEPs of children with disabilities. At that point, CCCC had several classrooms for younger students located in the Cedar Lane Unitarian Church, one of the few places that also housed a cooperative nursery school. The nursery school children entered the building through the same door and walked down the same hallway as the CCCC students. CCCC was on the left and the nursery school on the right. The two groups of children never played together on the playground or socialized in any way. In fact, the groups and their respective teachers had never met each other. The cooperative nursery school did not have a music program, so they were delighted to become part of the 1981 Special Project.

We integrated children from the two schools both ways. In the beginning I would bring one or two children from CCCC into the nursery school classroom for music. Then I would do the reverse. I shared music with the combined groups and also took them out onto the playground together to use the parachute or participate in other music and movement games. The beauty of this was that the children from both schools began to smile, wave, or say hello to each other. They would go out on the playground together, and the teachers started talking to one another.

I offered three different workshops for the parents of the children in the cooperative nursery school, explaining the objectives of the grant and how their children were serving as role models for the CCCC students. Later I presented additional workshops for both sets of parents together. It was really, really interesting… there were parents who met with me privately asking how this would work – long before the days of inclusive classrooms – and I had to allay their fears.

Part of the grant requirements included field-testing the curriculum, lesson plans, and individual music activities/experiences in other settings with mixed ages and populations. I wrote to many schools, clinics, and community centers offering music programs asking for their participation and input. Twenty-two sites in the Washington, DC area, a total of over 1,000 students between the ages of 2 and 22, were involved in the field-testing.

I designed evaluation forms for two separate groups of reviewers. This allowed me to improve the book's overall presentation as to its effectiveness, need, and format and include possible changes and appropriations/adaptations for use with populations with different needs from those enrolled in CCCC. Thanks to the input, expertise, and diligence of these educators and their students, *Target on Music* was recommended for use with children and adults with the following special needs: autism, deafness, deaf-blindness, emotional handicaps, hearing deficits, health impairments, mental retardation, multiple handicaps, orthopedic impairment, learning disabilities, speech and language impairments, and visual handicaps, as well as for young non-handicapped children. (This was the accepted terminology in 1981 for special populations.)

The grant funding paid for the research and the publication of the first edition of *Target on Music*. I was invited to speak at conferences about the project and the book. Many universities used it as a textbook then, as well as now, and I continue to enjoy the opportunity to participate in podcasts with college students enrolled as music therapy majors in today's changing world.

It was an extremely rewarding experience to create *Target on Music*, even though it required many hours and hard work! I usually do not enjoy doing research, but I was inspired by the challenge, knowing that the end result would be geared to practical, easily implemented music experiences for use in diverse settings. In addition, it filled an important educational void: integrating music interventions to enhance learning, specifically in the areas of motor development, communication, sensory integration, concept development, and social interaction.

Target on Music would never have been written without the input, guidance, experience, support, encouragement, and patience of Lillian Davis, assistant director of CCCC/Ivymount at that time, who meticulously added her educational expertise as my mentor/consultant/collaborator. Lillian empowered and motivated me, both in the classroom, and throughout our writing sessions. Our friendship has continued through the years, and I am eternally grateful for the many roles she has played in my life.

Many special people contributed to the book. Our photographer, Ruth Ephraim, was especially sensitive to our students, and it was heartwarming to learn, after the fact, that income received from her photos was used for the care of a handicapped sibling. Jane Putnam, our designer, knew little about music when she joined our team, but her graphics immediately captured the essence of the interventions, and she created beautiful illustrations of musical instruments, as well as carefully included musical notation for all the songs. Their assistance and encouragement were invaluable throughout *Target on Music's* creation, along with the support and generosity of all the staff, parents, and students in the CCCC/Ivymount community. Special thanks go to my husband and children for their patience and family involvement beyond the call of duty!

Did you hold the copyright for the book?

The Special Projects grant funding was awarded to the school, so they owned the copyright for the book. My role was as a "work for hire," but I held the copyright for all my original music.

Ivymount published the first edition of *Target on Music* in 1982. And, much to my, and the school's, amazement, there were requests for additional copies after these were sold. Also, many music therapists, music educators, and special education teachers had requested that I add more musical interventions and offered many excellent suggestions for a future publication. Thanks to the school's board of directors, a second edition, with a larger press run than the original, was published in 1988 giving me the opportunity to update, "fine tune," and expand the original publication, as well as for us to reformat and reinforce the book's physical structure.

When I retired from Ivymount after 30 years, (I finally graduated in 2005!), they gave me the copyright. Many people have asked if I would consider updating and publishing a third edition as the interventions are still being successfully used today, for which I am most grateful. However, with iTunes, the internet, YouTube, musical downloads, and continued developments in technology, many of the musical materials would need to be updated, as well as the addition of newer musical instruments, so I think I'll leave that to a future generation.

It seems like music therapy became an integral part of the Ivymount curriculum. How did that happen?

Music therapy became part of the students' Individual Education Plans (IEPs). I felt it was extremely important that music therapy be included in their IEPs, so I wrote music therapy goals and objectives for them. This meant if/when students left Ivymount to attend a different school, the IEP accompanied them, and their new teachers would know that the student possessed music abilities and that music therapy had contributed to educational outcomes. Maybe Johnny learned to cross the midline of his body by playing the xylophone. Because music is a motivator, a social skills builder, and a valuable tool for executive functioning, I felt this information was important to be embedded in his IEP. Some students are nonverbal but possess an excellent sense of rhythm and are able to express themselves musically even if they aren't singers/vocalists. With assistive technology, they are able to share their feelings and become more actively involved in musical experiences.

You never know the ripples that IEPs can create in a student's life. Many years ago, I worked with a five-year old boy and wrote music therapy goals in his IEP. He was one of those children who possessed perfect pitch. When he was playing the piano, he would ask, "Should I use my right or my wrong hand?" He knew the difference between right and left, and right and wrong, but he said "right or wrong hand" to be funny. Years later, I received a call from his social worker. Now in his late twenties, my former client was living in a group home. He wanted to have music lessons again, and the social worker found, through those old IEPs, that he had participated in music therapy sessions with me. It was very rewarding to reconnect and continue sharing/creating music with him in his adult years.

Another private music therapy client was able to use the strategies from our sessions to demonstrate that he could work in a community setting: listening and following directions, focusing on the task at hand, planning ahead, correcting mistakes, and completing assignments.

Another way that music therapy's role was expanded at Ivymount was through my increased collaboration with the therapists and special education staff. Working with the individual classroom teachers to integrate music therapy in their curriculum, e.g., history projects, science fairs, creative arts events, plays, and special programs, expanded the possibilities for music/music therapy with other learning.

In addition, I created several choral groups and with the speech/language, art teacher, and drama therapists we presented musicals throughout the year. We were also selected to perform at the Kennedy Center Very Special Arts, at Very Special Arts Festivals in Reston, VA, and for various community groups who were supporters of Ivymount School and its programs.

Do you have anything else to add to the story?

For my private music therapy clients, in the winter and spring, I held "Music Happenings" where those who wished to participate had the opportunity to share a song, solo, or musical duet, or reading with their family members, friends and other clients here in my studio, the very same room where their sessions were held, the only difference being the addition of extra chairs. These were very informal musical interludes, unlike the staged recitals and competitions I experienced during my school years. Although I prepared a printed program, the order was determined by the participants and frequently additional repertoire was spontaneously included at their request. Obviously, much encouragement, applause, and praise filled the room. These experiences helped them improve their self-esteem while highlighting what they had accomplished in a nourishing environment. Many clients later were able to participate in their school talent shows and performances in their communities.

I am extremely grateful that music therapy has helped define who I am and has allowed me to spread its voice! It has been a great honor and privilege for me to have been given countless opportunities to share the magic of music and music therapy experiences and interventions with so many wonderful children and adults, music educators, special education teachers, paraprofessionals, parents, and professionals and therapists in related fields over the years. I have learned and continue learning so much from all of them and am most grateful for the varied roles each of them has contributed to my life as we experienced, created, and shared music together! They never cease to enlighten and amaze me during every music therapy session. I've often been asked if I was tired of practicing music therapy as well as why I'm still working with children. As always, my answer remains what I said when I originally began my music therapy career, "I want to continue working with children, and when I grow up, I'll work with more adults."

WORKING WITH MULTIPLE CREATIVE ARTS THERAPIES

▶ by Paula Patterson

Paula Patterson, MA, RDT-BCT, is a creative arts therapist who has trained in many of the creative arts modalities and worked nationally and internationally. In addition to being credentialed as a registered drama therapist, she has trained extensively in Playback Theatre, psychodrama, sandtray therapy, and dance/movement therapy. While each modality focuses on a different aspect of the arts, there are many overlaps and ways that each can support the other. Her journey illustrates how creative arts therapists can work together and learn from each other, as well as how cross-training can broaden a creative arts therapist's abilities.

All creative arts therapists share the word "art." We each may be drawn to a specific discipline, but many of our techniques cross borders and feed each other. Many years ago, a national conference of all the creative arts therapies was held in Washington, DC. Creative arts therapists (CATs) did not go to attend workshops only on their own art form; they wanted to learn from each other! So many CATs gathered from across the US that they could not fit into the rooms assigned for the workshops.

My own experience with the creative arts therapies began when I chose to major in drama in college. "Whatever will you do with that?" my parents sniffed. By my senior year, I realized they may have been right. As much as I had always loved theater, I lacked the persona and extroversion to be comfortable in the cut-throat world of professional theater.

In my first years postgraduation, I worked a short stint as an airline stewardess and a longer one as an interior decorator for a prominent furniture store. At least I could wear costumes and play the role of a sophisticated designer or a sensual "Coffee, tea, or me?" stewardess. I also earned a license in practical nursing. After the required year postgraduation training in nursing, I specialized in psychiatric nursing. This was followed by marriage and an extended honeymoon in which I realized, "I don't want to work with what is on the outside of people: I want to work with what's inside of them."

Shortly before my wedding, I had learned of a progressive psychiatric hospital in which creative arts were an integral modality of the treatment. I interviewed the day after we returned home and was hired for the Activity Therapy department because of my combined background in drama, dance, and art. It's not that psychiatric hospitals were unwilling to hire a creative arts therapist back then, but they needed nurses, and stated, "When you're not involved in your nursing responsibilities, you can do that other stuff you like to do." I was invited to join the hospital's six-month "Social Therapy Program" in which we were introduced to multiple paradigms, and I was fascinated by the field of psychodrama, developed by Jacob Levy Moreno, MD.

Since certification and licensure weren't required in the 1970s, I simply introduced "Psychodrama Group" to our hospital. Its success led our medical director to offer me a six-month paid training at Moreno's Beacon Hill Institute in New York. I was overjoyed until complications in my first pregnancy required a difficult choice: I knew Dr. Moreno was dying, and I might not have another opportunity to study with him, but I could not allow the possibility of the death of my first child. I turned down the offer and continued my work at the hospital until the morning that not one, but two premature sons were born.

Three years later, I learned about drama therapy. However, the only creative arts therapy master's degree available in my city was dance/movement therapy. Now a wife and mother to three toddlers, it seemed impossible to relocate. I decided to apply for the first year that dance/movement therapy was offered as an MA program at Columbia College in Chicago.

I had always loved the joy and self-expression of movement. For my practicums and internship, I chose places that also used drama. A great blessing was to study with one of the pioneers of drama therapy, Marilyn Richman, at the Institute for Therapy through the Arts. I led groups in dance/movement therapy (where I quickly learned that having a hunky male coleader coerced guys to join the group), and one called "Sticky Situations." A common situation on the adolescent unit was a patient (the protagonist) facing their first "home pass" from the three-month in-patient program. They often anticipated that their former friends would invite them to "come party and get high with us." The adolescents loved playing the roles of the enticing friends and the psych patient hesitant to lose points toward discharge. "Changing roles" allowed them to "step into another's moccasins," as Moreno called it. Playing the role of the "double" (who speaks the unspoken words of the protagonist) developed insight in both the double and the protagonist.

When a workshop I planned to attend at the national psychodrama conference was cancelled, I chose another on Playback Theatre. I was enthralled with the concept of the playback actors listening with their hearts to a personal story by a teller related to the conductor or emcee of the group. The actors, chosen by the teller to play specific roles, would then play back not just the plot, but also the subtext they intuited the teller would wish to see. I signed up for the next one-week playback training led by its founder, Jonathan Fox, and continued through all levels of training.

At this point I had moved to San Diego, where my aging parents required care. There I founded and directed San Diego Playback Theatre. Having completed the alternate route to drama therapy registration, I worked as a registered drama therapist with Kaiser Permanente in a program for morbidly obese women. Our director allowed me to lead a group for women in the program who wished to engage in playback theatre. Stories of shame about their condition were empathically played back by their peers who truly understood the emotional consequences of obesity.

I felt great pride for some of the women in the Kaiser Permanente playback group, who agreed to be guest actors in the San Diego Playback Theatre. For most of them, it was the first time they did not allow their size to prevent them from appearing in public appearances or working with "normal-sized" playback actors.

While in San Diego, I married my current husband who was hoping to return to Florida, where he had been born. We agreed that we would do this when all three of my children were of college age. That time came, and we moved to Jacksonville, Florida. I implemented a drama therapy program at a private Integrative Medicine Program there. Learning there were other creative arts therapists in Jacksonville, I invited each of them to a meeting to discuss collaboration. The "Jax Cats" developed workshops in which participants could engage in all of the creative arts therapies. I only regret that at that time I was still unfamiliar about using many or all of the arts in the same experience to promote a profound as possible session. I also initiated "Playback Jax," and four of our eight actors attended the initial week of training at The School of Playback Theatre in New York.

A newspaper article about the drama therapy program I had initiated compared it to the arts in medicine program (AIM) at Shands Hospital of the University of Florida. Intrigued, my husband and I went to Gainesville to visit. We attended AIM's weekly Artist Rounds, where I was asked to demonstrate playback theatre. I did this with the aid of several willing artists.

At this time, I was enrolled in an MS program for mental health counseling through Nova Southeastern University. I used my one day off per week to commute to Shands as a volunteer for AIM. My title was "Dramatist in Residence" because at that time Shands was unwilling to employ creative arts therapists. Fortunately, they have seen the light, and creative arts therapists are now welcome.

I was offered a salaried position after two years, and my spouse and I moved to Gainesville, which I lovingly refer to as "the Berkeley of the swamp." For thirteen years, I worked at patient bedsides and directed performances throughout Shands/UF with family members, staff, and medical students.

I'll never forget the ill but rambunctious seven-year-old who led me on dramatic journeys that might start at the moon, shift to a mysteriously appearing MacDonald's, and end up with tickle fights on his bed. The younger the patient, the more I realized how important it was for them to take the lead. They could not challenge any of their doctors, nurses, or medical procedures, but for an hour per day, they could boss me around!

I began to train AIM artists of many disciplines in playback theatre. This became problematic, because every AIM artist wanted to be in the troupe, meaning that the other disciplines of art, music, dance and writing did not have available artists on Thursday afternoons when all were studying, rehearsing, and performing playback theatre. Therefore, we transitioned to mainly using volunteer actors from the community. We named ourselves "The Reflections," because our goal was to listen intensely to our patients' stories and reflect them back empathically. We used not only theater, but also dance and music in these spontaneous improvisations.

Some of our patients were with us in the hospital for over a year, if they awaited a new heart and were too medically unstable to wait at home. It was not unusual for a heart transplant patient to be summoned to the surgical unit while a donor heart was being rushed to the hospital only to learn after their surgical prep that the donor organ was not a good match or had an abnormality that prevented it from being used. In short, our heart transplant patients went on a wild ride of emotions, which they were able to express, then observe reflected back by Reflections actors either at their bedside or in a monthly performance for the whole floor. One patient decided in her second year of awaiting a heart that she wanted to join The Reflections and was graciously received by the other actors.

One Shands unit was for adolescents with diabetes whose families were unable to provide educational or emotional support on managing their disease. After returning to the hospital each day from a neighborhood school, the patients were taught how to measure their blood sugar levels, administer the proper amount of insulin to themselves, and be aware of complications. Before his retirement, a UF English professor had taught them theater games; I was brought in as his replacement. It was challenging to be accepted as a "dramatist," and not as a drama therapist. Although, I created treatment plans for each teen, I never wrote them in their charts. In AIM's weekly artist rounds, I would discuss the Teen Drama Troupe, when appropriate. I could request additional visits for a patient by an artist of a specific discipline (I might say to a musician-in-residence, "Patient A has started writing songs about his experience and brought his guitar in from home. Can I ask him if he would like for you to give him some musical pointers?"). At times, an artist might volunteer to work with a specific teen. When our Writer-in-Residence heard that a patient had started a journal, she offered to help her turn it into "Spoken Word."

AIM reaches out to the Gainesville Community. An administrator from the Harn Museum of Art shared her concern with me about an upcoming exhibition titled "The Culture of Violence." The previous year, our local community college had faced public outcry about a similar exhibition. Some locals felt it was condoning violence, rather than condemning it. I offered a suggestion to help address this issue, and it was approved by both the museum's board of directors and the director of AIM. Every AIM artist was eager to participate. On opening night, museum docents led small groups through the exhibit. AIM set up several tables where anyone could write or draw their reactions to the exhibit. They were then invited into the museum theater where we presented multi-media playback. All of the artists-in-residence were sitting in a semi-circle on stage, and anyone could rise after I had read or shown a participant's reaction. The playback to the comment might be offered through drama, dance, poetry, music, or song. Just as the AIM artists collaborated, and we all learned from one another, all creative arts therapies can support one another.

Having been drawn to doing relief work in Haiti after the 2010 earthquake, I initially worked on medical teams. Drama therapy was initiated by the survivors themselves. We once met in a clinic created by Engineers without Borders. A generator held up rubber walls. Somehow, one of the walls in the waiting area punctured, and the area collapsed. All of those waiting there ran out screaming, but the children who crept closer to investigate developed a game. "Get out, get out, the house is falling," they yelled, as they all ran out. They then ran back in and repeated the scenario. They did this multiple times, and I believe they were desensitizing themselves from traumatic earthquake memories.

Another time, just months post-earthquake, I was working in a physical therapy clinic. All the children were required to stay in the waiting room, so I decided my role was to keep them amused while their parents underwent treatment. I started with games using Emily Day's wonderful "Dancing Colors" scarves. At one point, one child picked up my whole array of scarves and initiated a process in which all the children chose to participate. Through complete improvisation, they all lay down, covered by all the scarves and chanted, "We are the dead, we are the dead." It was obvious to me that they were replaying the horror of seeing multiple bodies lying in the streets after the quake which claimed the lives of over 300,000 people. They did this over and over. There are times when our clients know what interventions they need, and our job, as creative arts therapists, is to be their witness.

On another medical trip, a throng of people brought in multiple survivors of a horrific car accident. They were followed by many children eager to see what happened. The children were crowding our physicians who were tending to the victims. A Haitian gentleman, who I had never met, quickly jumped in to assist me in drawing the children away through song and dance. Each child was given a 5 x 7 board and crayons. They completed their artwork while our doctors were attending the wounded. Not wanting them to rush back to crowd the physicians again, I started improvising a goofy theater and dance performance. Again, the Haitian gentleman quickly joined me. Even though we both spoke little of the other's language, intuition is an international language.

My most recent drama therapy experience was in supporting a theater improv teacher who had volunteered to work with seniors. Some of the seniors had left the class because they felt defeated by memory issues which deterred their full participation. I advocated for activities which were simple enough for them to feel successful. After we switched to this philosophy, all chose to remain. Creative arts therapists need to be attuned to the needs of whatever population we are serving. It is essential that we promote self-esteem with our clients.

My experience with AIM, where all the creative arts pollinated each other, reminded me of the importance of creative arts therapists sharing with one another. We all are passionate about healing through the arts. I have the least skill in music, but I can use a shaker egg and have the chutzpah to improvise a song. We don't have to be perfect in every creative art we use; we just need to be passionate about the use of the arts to promote healing.

I was delighted to recently receive an e-mail announcing an Expressive Arts Therapy Summit in Los Angeles. Workshops in creative arts therapies, including drama, dance, art, poetry, play, music, and sand tray will all be offered. Creative arts therapists have so much to share one with one another. After I studied sand tray therapy, I realized what a great warm-up it could be for a potential psychodrama. During a drama therapy group for morbidly obese women, one client could not articulate the challenges she experienced "being different." I asked if I could draw her outline on a large piece of butcher paper. I then gave her a variety of colored markers and asked her to first draw and then write what is inside a fat person. After she did that, she had a script she could refer to while walking across the room, gently touching the parts of herself she could not accept. This experiential process ended after I asked her to move or dance across the room, while adding a foot stomp to each touch. She did her best effort, and then broke into sobs. Several of the eight women in the group began to cry, as they shared how elements of her work had touched their own pain; for each of them felt different.

I wish to conclude by expressing the need for appropriate training: intuition and creativity are not enough. After completing the training to become a certified psychodramatist, I realized how much I had overlooked when I had led "Sticky Situations" with adolescents many years earlier.

There are only six accredited graduate schools of drama therapy in North America. However, not everyone realizes that there is also an alternate route to registration. I was lucky enough to have been mentored by board-certified trainer, Dr. Norman Fedder of Kansas State University. Because of the many similarities with dance/movement therapy, I was only required to take 3 courses in drama therapy before applying to NADTA for registration. There are many dedicated drama therapists who have applied to become a board-certified trainer. Any BCT will offer the same scholarly mentorship. ADTA also offers an alternate training program.

My 15 years with the arts-in-medicine program at Shands Hospital of the University of Florida demonstrated that cooperation among all the arts can only increase the power of each discipline. Let's work together!

MAKE LEMONADE OR GO THIRSTY: HOW I MANAGED GOING VIRTUAL

▶ by Jamie McCoppin

Jamie McCoppin, MA, RDT, is a registered drama therapist and founder of Spark of Play in New York City. She has spent the past 20 years honing her play skills through her creative work with groups and individuals from ages 3 to 100. Jamie is passionate about helping others reignite their spark, expand their range of self-expression, and increase their emotional intelligence to feel more joy and confidence in their everyday lives.

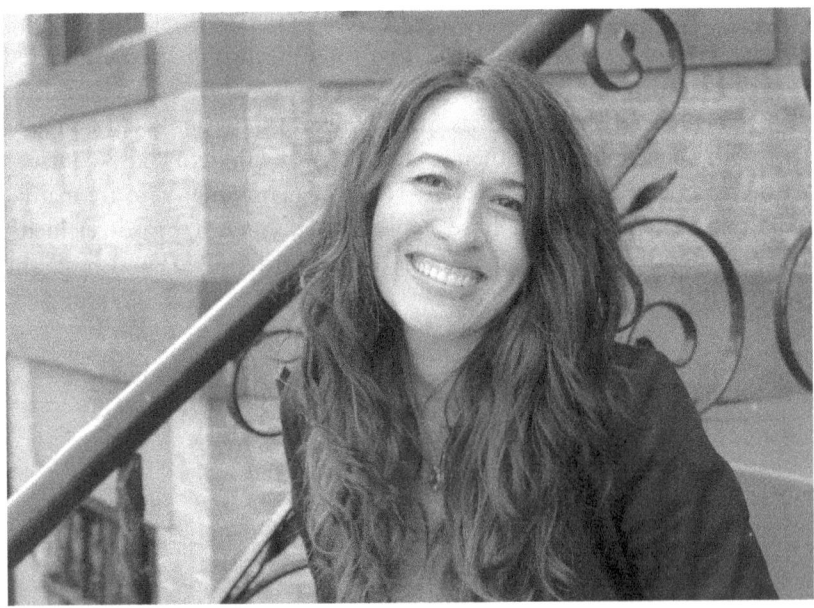

Figure 4.2 Jamie McCoppin, creator of "Spark of Play."

Introduction

Crisis requires creativity and a bit of humor. It was COVID versus the world, and, in my profession, it felt like COVID versus Creative Arts Therapists! The Covid-19 pandemic challenged us creative arts therapists to explore what was possible virtually. It's like the old saying, "When COVID pelts you with lemons, make lemonade, or go thirsty." Thank goodness imagination is a cornerstone of all the arts and a place where I feel at home. Imagination bridges the physical gap between us. And imagination helped me innovate in this complex time.

Spark of Play

After majoring in Media Communications, I spent a number of years working as an after-school teacher, a babysitter, an ABA line therapist, a hospital clown, a birthday party entertainer, and a substitute teacher, before going to graduate school for drama therapy. After that, I worked in a senior home, a pediatric hospital, and for the Post Traumatic Stress Center, in the public schools of New Haven and in their outpatient trauma clinic.

As a drama therapist with a focus in personal growth and development, I had just started my private coaching business in April 2019 in New York City. I was building the brand for "Spark of Play," but I wasn't sure who I specifically wanted to help. Why not help everyone? But that's not how a successful business works, said my business coach. (Cue sad trombone sound, "Womp-womp.")

Nevertheless, I indulged in experimenting with different workshops, exploring various "ideal clients." In other words, I was throwing a lot of spaghetti on the wall to see what stuck. Simply choosing a niche without exploration felt agonizing to me since I believe everyone needs play in their life.

Taking great delight in my "spaghetti on the wall" approach, I created workshops for stuck creatives, workshops for teachers on how to bring more play and joy into their classrooms, workshops for corporate teams wanting stress relief, and more. I was out on the town many nights of the week networking at events with various NYC social communities interested in personal growth and development. Among them, I became known as the "play expert," but my business was still slow to take off that first year. I noticed most grown-ups considered "play" to be frivolous or, at best, saw my services as a luxury they couldn't afford or prioritize, even when I hosted free or by-donation playshops. However, that attitude was about to change when everything in our lives changed with the COVID-19 virus, and play became less of a luxury and more of a need.

Before mainstream awareness of the virus took hold in New York City, I was feeling energized around three projects I had cooking: *Playing It Real, Out of Your Comfort Zone*, and *PLAYdating NYC*. Many hours were poured into the creation and facilitation of these projects in addition to a small caseload of private coaching clients I saw on a weekly basis.

Playing It Real

In *Playing It Real: A Workshop Series to Build Social Confidence*, I used sociodrama as a holding structure to explore all sorts of social anxieties like online dating, public speaking, and attending events alone just to name a few. Sociodrama is an action method developed by J.L. Moreno in which the group votes on a shared group issue or challenge to be explored using role play and improvisation (Sternberg and Garcia, 2000). The first *Playing It Real* cohort had successfully completed the program a few months earlier in October 2019.

On March 11, 2020, the third cohort had its last meeting in person before the lockdown. That evening, only one of the participants opted to stay home. The rest of us agreed to no physical contact and lots of hand sanitizing. As part of our warm-up, we created unique new ways of greeting one another in place of the traditional handshake or high five.

Out of Your Comfort Zone

Out of Your Comfort Zone was a new 1:1 coaching program I had dreamed up for young professionals in New York who wanted to be more playful, more spontaneous, more flexible and to "get out of their comfort zone." I had heard this phrase repeatedly over the previous year in different communities who all shared the desire for social connection and personal growth in some way.

In *Out of Your Comfort Zone*, I planned to use a particular drama therapy method I have extensive training in, called Developmental Transformations (DvT). This method differs from other drama therapy methods in that the therapist and the client mutually agree to enter a "playspace," where everything that transpires is created together based on portraying real or imagined beings and situations (Johnson, 2009). Being in the playspace can often feel like a lucid dream where the client and therapist play with dramatic images as they come up or likewise discard them creating a non-linear experience using sound, movement, physicality, and roles. Another unique aspect of this method is that it usually takes place in a bare room with some carpeting and pillows. What remains is just you and the other or, in some cases, a group of others.

The first sessions were set to begin Tuesday, March 10. Each encounter looked very different but left me feeling energized and joyful. The play I shared with each participant felt natural and easy from my point of view. Each encounter was highly physical, and, in one case, there was full body contact with a participant who had experience with Contact Improvisation. It's also important to mention here that physical contact in DvT is discussed prior to the session and defined in the contract ensuring all physical touch is appropriate to the play itself and non-sexual in nature.

By our first session on March 10, there was some rising awareness about the coronavirus, but I fell into the "I feel healthy, and as long as I am washing my hands, I'm not worried" camp. Well, March 10th was our first and last session where that was even a possibility!

PLAYdating NYC

PLAYdating had always been intended to be experienced in a *physical* space where singles could connect through play, art, humor, movement, and imagination. We had started to build a following with our wildly fun three-hour events that included several creative arts components, a guest speaker on dating and relationships, and, of course, lots of drama games that often resulted in laughter and, sometimes, a love connection.

Little did I know that Thursday, March 12 would be the last day I left my neighborhood for the next three months, the last day I would ride the subway for the next six months, and the last time I would work with people in the same physical space for more than a year. My anxious thoughts raced, "What about my programs? What will happen to my livelihood? I'm a drama therapist! My work is all about physical embodiment! How will I survive?" New York City rent is not cheap. They even wrote a Broadway musical about this issue you may have heard about. It's called *Rent*.

Through my panic during the first day of lockdown, we decided to make our PLAYdating event virtual. I'll admit, it was awkward! I had never tried conducting drama games over Zoom before, and I did not anticipate how much more energy it took me to hold space and model playfulness through the screen! The flow of the games was definitely off, but I soon became aware of the new shape and form of the event as it was unfolding.

Afterwards, one participant commented that they enjoyed the discussion on love and dating more than the games. The discussion arose from a modified "Spectrogram." Typically, I used Spectrograms in a physical space where participants placed themselves on an imaginary scale from 1 – 10 across the room in response to different quotes or statements. For Zoom, I had them hold up their fingers to indicate where they "stood" on the imaginary line. This one was a keeper, whereas the storytelling game, "Fortunately, Unfortunately" fell on its face when participants were confused about who was supposed to go next. It wasn't until months later when I figured out that one way to alleviate this problem would be to make the order clear by numbering participants with the 'Renaming' feature on Zoom.

My *Playing It Real* group was, for the most part, game to moving our meeting to Zoom. My fabulous NYU drama therapy intern and I created modifications to sociodrama in one afternoon that we taught to the group that evening. Suddenly, we were a group of talking heads. How could I get them up and moving around? What became quite apparent that first night on Zoom was a shared need to talk and connect around what was really happening – the fears and uncertainty of our world being turned upside down. Our hustle and bustle New York City lifestyle had been halted practically overnight. We were in shock. It was a time for me, as the leader, to let go of the agenda in service of the group.

We did find our way to play over the following few weeks. In some ways, individuals demonstrated more confidence in their roles and characters, taking more risks than ever before. What had changed? Something we introduced in this new virtual experience was costuming. Being a drama therapist in NYC without a vehicle, I never considered schlepping a bag of costume pieces with me all over the city. But the convenience and novelty of everyone having their own closet full of potential costumes from their own home worked in our favor. I would give participants just a few minutes on the timer to go and find something in their closet to help define their characters. This brought a fresh wave of silliness to the group and allowed for more permission to try out new ways of talking and using their voices as well.

My *Out of Your Comfort Zone* participants were also game to trying Zoom. This was the first time I had done virtual DvT. The use of the camera was a game-changer the day I realized we could pick up our devices and move around the room, fall on the floor, get down low, etc. The camera became another participant in the play. On a suggestion from my DvT supervisor, Navah Steiner, we tried using a different structure: after about 20 minutes of play, we would turn off our cameras and free write about the experience in a journal. I invited the participant to think of it as spontaneous poetry if they chose or to simply list the images and themes that stayed with them from the encounter that just occurred. After five minutes, we would turn our cameras back on and read our poems/reactions to each other. This was a closing structure that worked well and also gave us a chance to process a bit of the play together. This was a sharp turn from classic DvT, but then again, 2020 has been one big sharp turn, so it seemed fitting.

Play+Ground

It had been a few years since I had worked with children in a clinical capacity, because when I turned 40, I made a firm decision to focus my energy on supporting adults. But the world had just been turned upside down, and I clearly saw a way I could pitch in.

So, one sleepless night, I got up and wrote down the vision for a way to help kids during this uncertain time. The name of the program would be *Play+Ground*. We would check-in around our feelings. We would dance, draw, play… and ground with a simple grounding technique. Kids needed a place to connect, create, and calm down. I could provide a simple holding structure where they could share and process their feelings about what was happening through various creative arts activities.

After a few phone calls with mothers and a couple of Facebook posts about the program, I was hosting as many as five *Play+Ground* groups per week starting in April 2020. The program continued to grow through word of mouth. Several parents told me their child was resistant to all other offerings online, but when it came to Play+Ground, they counted down the days.

The magic sauce of *Play+Ground* was in keeping a playful, spontaneous self-expressive atmosphere that virtual school classrooms were most likely unable to allow. I found that beginning with a dramatic structure or a game and allowing the structure to break was key. I'll never forget one of the first magical moments this happened on its own.

I was playing a game called "TV Channels" with a group of eight- and nine-year-olds. I directed everyone to turn off their videos unless I called on them. I started off as the narrator saying things like, "We take you to the Spanish Cooking Channel," or "Show me the Sports Channel!" At one point, I blurted out, "We take you to the Doctor's Channel" before I even considered the fact that the little girl's mother was a pediatric doctor who was still working through the pandemic. There was a moment of hesitation before the girl (let's call her Emily), said, "Hold on a minute, I have to go get my mask!" When Emily walked away from her computer, at that point, the structure naturally broke. I took a risk, and the kids followed my lead. I said, "I think Emily needs help. Who wants to play the nurse? Who wants to play the patient?" The kids knew exactly what to do and started volunteering for different roles. The energy was high as we were talking about something very real… the nurse was frantic, trying to save the dying patients in the hospital waiting room. Emily finally returned as the doctor and said it was time for her lunch break and pretended to eat a sandwich. This provided some comic relief as Amelia, the nurse, was on her own to help the suffering patients.

In another group with five- and six-year-olds, we pretended to go to Florida and swim in a pool together. It wasn't long before one little girl pretended she was drowning. I called on someone to rescue her. Someone else saw a shark in the pool. The drama continued to heighten! At the end of the group, I learned that for the entire group, our "drowning" participant hadn't been able to see any of us because she was having video trouble! But she could hear us, so she continued to participate! This was illuminating to me because I realized that the shared imagination was so strong that we were all still able to engage in the story we were creating on the spot. That is, we all had our eyes closed and still had a blast.

One of my groups of seven-year-olds started a silly ritual of renaming themselves ridiculous names, knowing that I would call them by whatever they wrote each time with a straight face, even if it was a bunch of consonants strung together. One time the entire group renamed themselves my name. So, I'd call on Jamie McCoppin, and they'd say, "Which one?" Who knew that my clown training in playing the fool would help build group confidence?

Virtual backgrounds and video filters on Zoom are very theatrical! I might invite the group to create characters or a story together using these devices.

Once I allowed a group of 10-year-old girls to check-in with a virtual background that matched how they were feeling that day.

Besides the obvious safety issues, kids are getting savvy on Zoom, distracted by all of its cool features. One is the disappearing act where they walk away from their camera or turn their video off. A rule I have had to implement in Play+Ground is to "stay on camera, otherwise we spend all of our time worrying about what happened to you instead of playing together!"

The beauty of leading groups online is witnessing the friendships and connections that can form all across the country and the world. One day I'd like my *Play+Ground* groups to include children from different parts of the world sharing and connecting about their daily experiences through the universal language of play.

As we move into the future, I would like to continue to support others remotely as much as possible. In addition to my *Play+Ground* program, my individual caseload has tripled in the pandemic as more and more adults are seeking play for healing in their lives. Body intelligence is another big focal point in my work, and I appreciate how individuals can feel less inhibited tuning into themselves while in their own private spaces on the other side of the screen. Of course, I miss seeing the whole person. I feel the impairment the most in DvT. The inability to see the whole body leaves out a lot of information. I also miss the physical contact that can be very healing in the DvT playspace.

I believe my imagination has strengthened in this time. There's no doubt that I am missing things like body language displayed off screen, for instance, but missing things is inevitable during in-person work as well. There has been a special permission in this time to experiment as a virtual creative arts therapy pioneer. This permission has allowed me to relax around the inherent imperfection of the virtual medium and discover new, unexpected possibilities – like the day I picked up my laptop and spun around the room. So, cheers to you, 2020, you rascal. I am enjoying my big glass of COVID lemonade. Even if it is only pretend, I'll keep drinking it.

References

Johnson, D. R. (2009). Chapter 6: Developmental transformations: Toward the body as presence. In D. R. Johnson & R. Emunah (Eds.). *Current approaches in drama therapy.* (2nd ed., pp. 89–112). Charles C. Thomas.

Sternberg, P., & Garcia, A. (2000). *Sociodrama: Who's in your shoes?* Praeger.

CHAPTER 5

STARTING AGAIN

Sally Bailey, Loretta Gallo-Lopez, Azizi Marshall, Kevin Spencer, Michelle Yadon, Tracena Marie, Mizuho Kanazawa, Barbara McKechnie, and Randy Mulder

Introduction

There are times in a career when an unexpected coincidence changes the direction of one's path. The creative arts therapists whose essays are in this chapter have been called to explore new directions. However, even in these new endeavors, they are using every bit of skill and expertise they developed in their careers as CATs.

Loretta Gallo-Lopez was called upon by parents of her adolescent clients to establish a safe, nurturing place for them to learn, using all the arts educationally and therapeutically. She stepped up to the challenge and founded a private high school for students with neurodifferences.

Azizi Marshall dreamed of being an entrepreneur and creating a Center for Creative Arts Therapy where everyone could come and experience the joy and healing that the arts can provide.

Kevin Spencer left a career as a magician to bring magic into special education classrooms as an educational tool and to survivors of trauma in many parts of the world.

Two drama therapists, Michelle Yadon and Tracena Marie, report on how they worked to expand their practices and the practices of their fellow CATs by

DOI: 10.4324/9781003035664-5

advocating for creative arts therapies to be included in the Medicaid waiver in their state of Indiana.

Mizuho Kanazawa and Barbara McKechnie share the saga of the NJ Task Force for Drama Therapy and Dance/Movement Therapy as they advocated their state legislators to pass licensure for all the creative arts therapists in their state. Together, the members of the task force began a long journey of learning about legislation, how state governments create and pass laws, and how compromise is an inevitable part of politics.

Randy Mulder became captivated by Playback Theatre, an applied theater method that can be used for community entertainment, social justice work, and drama therapy. His commitment grew to the point that he created a non-profit theater: Village Playback Theatre, located in New York City, providing educational and therapeutic outreach to schools and organizations in the city and environs. Here he shares the tale of how, under the auspices of a grant from the National Endowment for the Arts, he and his troupe addressed the stigma of mental illness through playback.

FOCUS ACADEMY: CREATING CONNECTION AND EQUALIZING EDUCATION THROUGH THE ARTS

▶ by Loretta Gallo-Lopez

Loretta Gallo-Lopez, MA, LMHC, RDT-BCT, RPT-S, is a founder and clinical director of Focus Academy, an innovative high school and transition program for students with significant cognitive and developmental disabilities. She is co-editor of the books *Play Therapy with Adolescents* and *Play Based Interventions for Children and Adolescents with Autism Spectrum Disorders*.

The arts enable each of us to create in our own way, to express who we are, what we love, what we believe, and to give life to our dreams. To me it seems quite natural to design a school for young people with developmental and cognitive disabilities that relies on the limitless power and boundless possibilities of the arts and creative imagination, to establish a more equitable learning environment and expand the opportunities for students who have been traditionally marginalized and limited by systemic barriers.

In 2010, a small group of parents in Tampa, Florida came to me to share concerns about their children's current educational environments which were not providing a positive experience or the level of success they saw their children demonstrating in the ACT after-school drama therapy project I was leading. They felt strongly that drama therapy should be the cornerstone of a new high school designed specifically to address their children's academic and personal success. They wanted me to be part of the planning and to play a role in administering the school. Focus Academy became the embodiment of that dream. Over the past 10 years, I've come to realize that Focus Academy had probably been part of my dream for years before that; I just hadn't realized it until the parents made the offer. I've been saying, "Yes, and..." ever since.

When I was an aspiring young actress, I began working as a special education teacher in a New York City public school. It was perfect: I had a steady paycheck, great hours, my summers off. My degree was not in education, so I did what I knew. Having facilitated theater groups for children and teens in camps and after-school programs while in college, I relied on those experiences to teach my students all the basics and more through dramatic play and other hands-on creative arts experiences. My students made costumes and puppets, created scenery, painted murals, and acted out historical events. They drew self-portraits and became superheroes. In the process they learned academic and social skills required by the curriculum. I couldn't put my finger on it, but I knew there was something special, almost magical, about how my special education students were responding to all this creativity.

By the autumn of my third year of teaching, my students were regularly utilizing the arts as a learning tool, a means of self-expression, and a pathway to growth and understanding. These were still students with tremendous challenges and significant behaviors, but they were able to focus, sit calmly, and listen to each other. The week before Thanksgiving, they were excited to share an in-class performance for several other classes, staff members, and our program administrator. Dressed as Native Americans, their faces beamed as they proudly sang their songs, beating out the rhythm on their drums. Everyone applauded, and they joyfully bowed together, but the only comment from our program administrator was, "Why aren't they wearing their shoes?" A defining moment for me, and six simple words I have never forgotten. I knew that the work I had been doing had power and meaning, but I also realized that, unfortunately, this school was not where I was meant to do this work.

That very afternoon I made the short, determined trip to NYU to pick up their latest course catalogue. I opened it up and saw: Introduction to Drama Therapy. I wasn't exactly sure what drama therapy was, but once I read the course description, I knew that this was what I was meant to do. I was going to be a drama therapist.

I worked with children and adolescents as a registered drama therapist in a variety of interesting and inspiring settings. After several years, I left the burgeoning and exhilarating creative arts therapy community of New York City for Tampa, Florida, where drama therapy was virtually unheard of.

After several years in Tampa, I started a private practice where I continued to use drama therapy with children and adolescents, including those who had experienced significant trauma. Additionally, because of my background in special education, colleagues often referred children, teens, and young adults with developmental and cognitive disabilities to my practice. I developed a sub-specialty: A significant focus of my practice was working with children and teens with autism. I worked closely with their schools, did regular student observations, attended individual education plan (IEP) meetings, and assisted school staff in developing behavior plans in the hopes of helping my clients to have more successful school experiences. Many of these young people with autism were struggling due to deficits in social competency. "Maria," a middle school girl with autism, kept getting in trouble for giving unwanted hugs to girls at her school whom she didn't know. Ultimately, she was suspended, and the school began to express concern that she might be a sexual predator. Via role play during one of our therapy sessions, it became obvious that Maria was merely copying what she saw other middle school girls doing – hugging friends at the start and end of each school day. Due to her lack of social awareness and her need to fit in, she was mimicking behavior that she clearly didn't understand. As Maria was not part of that friend group, her hugs were unwanted. We worked through role play and improvisation to help Maria understand about different types of relationships and the basic rules of social interaction.

Mimicking the social behavior of other students at school was the basis of many of the problems my young clients with autism experienced. Their lack of social communication and social interaction skills made middle school and high school a lonely and torturous experience. This was obviously a very significant problem that was not being addressed.

In 2006, in response to this significant need, I started the All Community Theatre (ACT) Project. The ACT Project began as a drama therapy program for 8 – 12-year-olds with an autism spectrum disorder diagnosis. The hope was that by helping children develop important social and communication skills during this crucial time in their lives, they would be better prepared to tackle the social dilemmas that would lie ahead. Groups met once a week after school for 90 minutes throughout the school year. The goal of the program was to provide participants an opportunity to improvise and work together to create characters and develop scripts based on their interests and passions. Through warm-up exercises participants began the work of enhancing social awareness and practicing essential skills to strengthen their sense of social competence and connection. Sharing scenes and stories they had created with their family and friends via performance became an integral part of the program and an important way for ACT participants to further enhance their connection to others and their level of social ease and comfort. Group members formed friendships, and the work of the groups enabled participants to experience progress as they practiced important social skills in a safe and supported environment.

I soon partnered with fellow drama therapist, Lisa Powers. Together we expanded the program, adding teen groups and serving a broader population, including individuals with other developmental and cognitive disabilities. Our participants looked forward each week to their group sessions, which were fun, creative, and joyful. Parents began noticing significant improvements in their children's overall well-being, self-confidence, and in their ability to interact and connect with others.

In 2010, that small group of ACT Project parents came to ask me to spearhead the establishment of Focus Academy for their children, a school where their children's academic and social needs would be primary. I was inspired by the idea and immediately agreed without ever thinking about the immense amount of work that would be involved or the fact that none of us had ever attempted anything like this before. I was invigorated by the challenge and by what we could accomplish. Many of the students we would serve were capable of much more than they were demonstrating at their current schools. Many were stalled and had made little-to-no progress in years. Our fundamental guiding purpose was and continues to be that our students would not just make academic improvements but would experience dramatic growth and life-long positive change. We knew that what we built would need to be groundbreaking and address all of the failings of the schools currently serving this population of students. With the understanding that a sense of connection, of being part of a school community, has a significant positive impact on students' overall school experiences, strengthening our students' sense of connection and belonging became the essence and the heart of all that we would do at Focus Academy.

Focus Academy opened its doors in August 2013 with 26 students. Our new school served students ages 14 – 22, diagnosed with significant cognitive and/or developmental disabilities, such as autism and Down syndrome. Every attempt was made to ensure that this was a more positive school experience for each of our students. With that goal in mind, a half-day event which we called our "Field Day" was scheduled several days before the first day of school to enable students to begin to get to know one another, their teachers, and their new school. Our goal was to minimize student anxiety related to the first day at a new school by providing students an opportunity to spend a few hours together having fun. In small groups, students played getting-to-know-you and other warm-up games using art and drama activities and large colorful beach balls. Students enjoyed playing, creating, and socializing. We knew when they returned for the first day

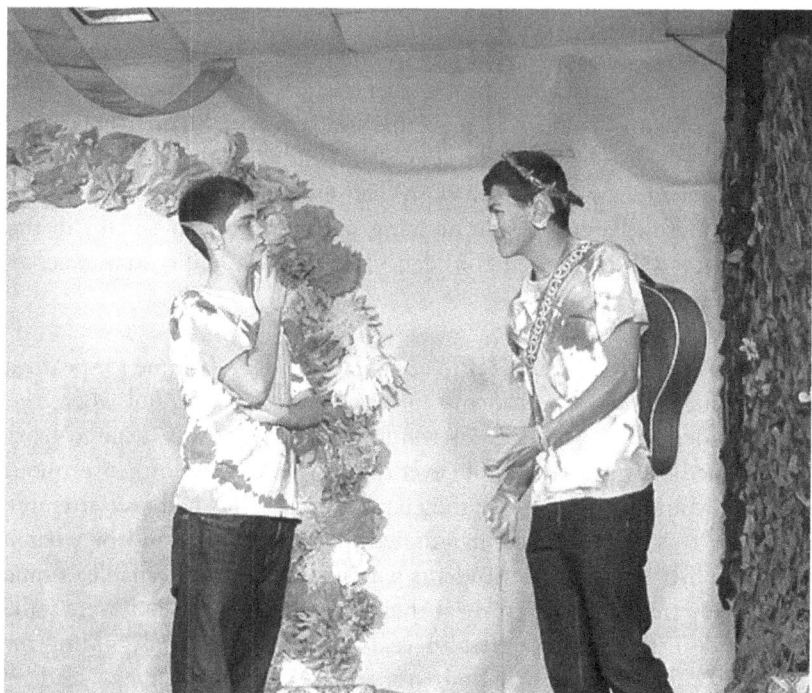

Figure 5.1 Students perform at Focus Academy.

of school they would be returning to a place where they already felt at home. There was very little anxiety the first day of school. Since then, Field Day has become an annual event, enabling returning and new students to get to know each other, play games, sing karaoke, create art together, and reduce the anxiety related to the start of a new school year.

Every day at Focus Academy begins with Morning Meeting, where all students and staff come together to experience a sense of community and celebration. Accomplishments and special days are celebrated, Words of Wisdom are shared, and to enhance students' understanding of humor, students take turns telling jokes, all with the goal of preparing everyone for the day ahead.

Focus Academy students participate in small group drama therapy at least twice per week. In addition, the philosophical perspective of connection and belonging that underlies our drama therapy programming is infused throughout the school day and within our overall school climate. Drama interventions include activities that focus on building verbal and non-verbal communications skills, such as reading and responding to body language and facial expression, use of vocal tone, and reciprocal conversation skills. Using our collection of old phones, students practice reciprocal conversation skills such as attentive listening, asking and responding to questions, and using appropriate greetings. By exploring and experimenting with a wide variety of roles, students learn to problem solve, envision a wider array of options, and break through rigid behavior patterns to develop new and more functional behaviors and responses. Via drama therapy, our students improvise and work together to create and develop scripts based on individual and shared interests. Dance, music, and art experiences help to further develop characters and stories. By creating and working together to incorporate individual character and story ideas into a cohesive whole, students learn to collaborate, negotiate, and compromise. They learn and practice empathy skills, developing an appreciation for the perspective of others. Via role play, improvisation, and performance, students build processing speed, working memory, focus and concentration, self-confidence, active listening, self-regulation, and collaborative problem-solving skills. Group drama therapy provides social learning experiences that serve to inspire and support creative imagination, enabling our students to reach deep within themselves, defying conventional expectations.

Students participate in several performances each year. For many of our students their first Focus Academy performance may be the first time they have ever performed in front of an audience. It is always exhilarating – and often life-changing. Performance allows students to share what they have created and allows others to bear witness to the process and product of their work developed via collaboration and creative imagination. Performance serves to build on and enhance the sense of a shared experience. As a result of these experiences, our students have become not just more successful learners, but more socially competent, connected, and engaged members of their community.

As our students can remain at Focus Academy until the year they turn 22, we have established a Transition Program for students who have completed 12th grade. The transition program is designed with the same focus on social connection and relationship building but with a specific emphasis on employability and life skills. Drama therapy groups use role play for a variety of purposes ranging from exploring relationship dilemmas and social expectations to practicing job interviews and workplace behaviors. Students focus on exploring future goals and experimenting with various roles and situations via improvisation.

Focus Academy continues to grow as a school, and our students consistently demonstrate progress. We currently serve approximately 110 students via our 9th – 12th grade and Transition programs. Although the growth of a school is indicative of at least some level of success, Focus Academy intentionally has limited growth as our model is based on a somewhat small student population. Our maximum student population will be approximately 150 students.

Measurable success, however, can be determined and described in a variety of ways. Most traditionally we look at academic success, including reading and math levels and graduation rates. Likely as a result of our intensive focus on building social competency, we typically see a significant improvement in this area in a student's first year at Focus Academy, followed by consistent progress over subsequent years. This is measured by observation and annual parent and teacher surveys. Most notably, however, our data shows that, for a majority of our students, an improvement in social skills is followed by between one half to up to two years' improvement annually in both reading and math levels. This is especially significant given that the majority of our students begin Focus Academy as high schoolers reading at between a kindergarten and third-grade level, with many having made no progress at all in many years. We continue to collect data and are consistently seeing that an intense and deliberate focus on strengthening social competency skills appears to lead to significant academic gains.

As far as graduation rates, Focus Academy has graduated over 80 students in the past six years. Our current graduation rate is 94.4%. In comparison, the state of Florida's current graduation rate for traditional students is 86.8% and the graduation rate for special education students is 79.7%.

I also measure success by noting the acceptance and recognition of drama therapy within and outside of our school community. Everyone from our board of directors to our parents and staff clearly understand and openly discuss the benefits of drama therapy and detail how positively students have been impacted by this approach. Drama therapy is written into every student's IEP – a legal document – as the primary intervention used to support social-emotional growth, self-regulation, social skill development, and emotional health and well-being.

We could easily measure success by examining the progress of individual students. There are as many wonderful stories of individual successes at Focus Academy as there are students. Jenny's story is one that stands out because of her uniqueness and the swiftness with which growth occurred. Jenny is a student with autism. Jenny first showed us what she was capable of through music. Like the majority of Focus Academy students, Jenny had never performed on stage before, and, although she loved to sing, she had never been in front of an audience. She sang only at home in her mirror along with her favorite YouTube videos. Her ASD symptoms are significant and, throughout her life, have negatively impacted her ability to interact with others and to see any true level of success in a school environment. When she first began at Focus, she scripted and repeatedly screamed words and phrases over and over again, engaged in a great deal of repetitive body movement such as rocking and pacing, was rigid and ritualistic in her behaviors, and, when not gaining negative attention by putting her hands on other students, tended to isolate herself from others.

The first time Jenny stood on the stage in music class, microphone in hand, she began to sing a Disney princess song. She knew every word and sang beautifully, engaging the audience with such intensity and passion that her peers jumped to their feet in applause, and the staff were brought to tears. She would sing often and always as beautifully. She loved the applause and began to look forward to the positive attention of her peers. In her drama therapy groups she enjoyed taking on characters and interacting with peers in short scenes. Within a few months, staff began to notice improvement in her ability to manage her behavior and to work successfully in her academic classes. Teachers recognized that she was able to read and successfully work at a level much higher than she had previously been thought capable of. During performances, she amazes our audiences with her singing and her ability to fully play characters, expressing emotion and demonstrating reciprocity as she engages in scenes with her fellow actors. The more she performs, the more progress she seems to make in her ability to appropriately interact with peers, to communicate her thoughts and feelings, and to begin to build relationships. Jenny is, of course, still a student with autism, scripting, rocking, sometimes yelling, but she is also experiencing success, demonstrating greater social competence, and becoming a more connected and happier member of the world around her. Without a doubt – immeasurable success.

CREATING YOUR OWN CREATIVE ARTS THERAPY BUSINESS

▶ by Azizi Marshall

Azizi Marshall, MA, LPC, RDT-BCT, REAT, is the founder & CEO of the Center for Creative Arts Therapy, an arts-based psychotherapy practice and training center in Chicago, which has launched such programs and companies as Psychology Arts, Arts Playschool, Artful Wellness, and the Therapeutic Performance Initiative model. She has been featured in Oprah Magazine, Thrive Global, CNN, NBC News, Bustle, Reader's Digest, The Huffington Post, Chicago Tribune, and Glancer Magazine. She speaks regularly throughout the country on Creative Arts Therapy, and guest posts on national news articles about wellness and creativity.

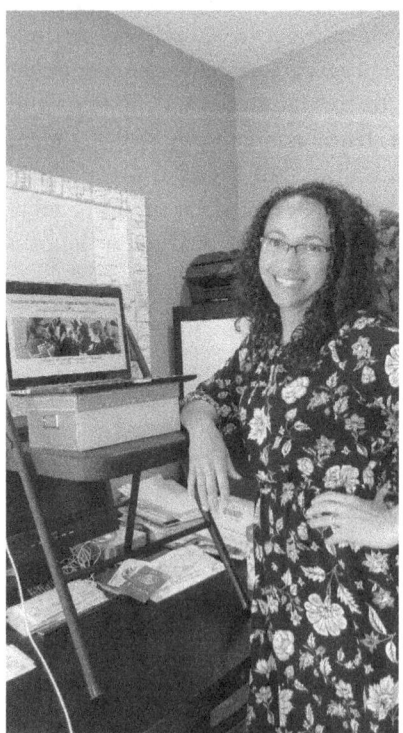

Figure 5.2 Creative arts therapist Azizi Marshall at the Center for Creative Arts Therapy, Downer's Grove, IL.

Introduction

I am the founder & CEO of the Center for Creative Arts Therapy, a full-service, arts-based psychotherapy practice and training center. It is dedicated to nourishing emotional wellness and expression through the arts and allowing clients to explore the arts in a comfortable, non-judgmental environment. The Center for Creative Arts Therapy provides visual arts, movement, drama/improvisation, music, and writing to help clients discover, accept, and express themselves and use the arts as a new way to tap into their true selves and to connect with others on the same path.

We offer support groups for first responders, teenagers, children, and young adults. We also offer a therapeutic theater program, where we create original theatrical performances that express participants' personal stories through dance, music, and storytelling. They are the creators, directors, and performers. While it is hard to pick one group over another, the one I get the most energy from is our therapeutic theater program. During one of our projects at an all-girls high school, we created an original musical based on their lives. The Illinois High School Theatre Association was so impressed by what we had done, that they invited us to be the first student-led workshop in their history. It was an empowering experience for those girls, and some have presented with me again at other conferences on how theater is therapeutic.

The Center for Creative Arts Therapy's international training center offers classes and training that lead toward a Registered Drama Therapist and/or a Registered Expressive Arts Therapist credential. Our classes are specifically customized for our students' interests and include Expressive Arts Therapy with War Veterans, Drama Therapy for Eating Disorders, Multi-Modal Arts Integration, and Therapeutic Theatre.

One of our programs, Arts Playschool, is an arts-based social-emotional learning platform for children ages 3 – 7 and their parents. We have recently created an online membership model for families to learn how to raise resilient and enlightened children through videos, live classes, and parent resources containing meditations, creative movement, music, cultural crafts, and stories.

The Center for Creative Arts Therapy is the Award Recipient of Excellence in Creative Dramatics by the Illinois Theatre Association. I have been featured on CNN, Oprah Magazine, Reader's Digest, Huffington Post, Thrive Global, The Sun Times, My Suburban Life, Glancer Magazine, and the Chicago Tribune for my work in healing communities through the arts.

I love what I do. Here's how I got there.

Early Beginnings

Growing up in a household of two artistic psychotherapist parents, I learned at an early age that people are beautifully complex. I was witness to how the arts could guide extremely troubled individuals and communities to a place of healing and growth. I observed my father transform his clients from people who hated life to people who loved themselves. It was not through traditional talk therapy but through a therapeutic intervention called psychodrama: the marrying of psychotherapy and theater.

My upbringing was far from normal, yet it was my normal. Whenever my family and I would have a disagreement or familial challenge, we would act it out using psychodrama. One day, my father told my brother and me that we were going to be the parents for the morning, and he was going to be the child. Our mission was to get my dad ready for school and in the car. My brother and I looked at one another and simultaneously thought, "No problem." Well, after several hours of my father playing with his food, running around the house, distracting himself with the television, forgetting multiple items inside (such as his lunch, backpack, jacket, and shoes), we finally got him in the car.

My brother and I were exhausted as we closed the doors to the car with my father buckled in the back seat. With a distinctive smirk on my father's face, he asked us, "So… how was that?" My brother and I groaned in dismay, as we then knew we now had to process the scene. After further exploration on the many ways we, as the parents, struggled to get our "child" in the car, we came to realize that his behaviors were similar to the behaviors we had engaged in while getting ready for school each day.

The next day, our father found my brother and me standing by the back door, having eaten breakfast, ready with our backpacks, lunches in hand, and jackets and shoes on. A successful psychodrama had been accomplished within our home, one that opened our eyes to the struggles our parents went through each and every school day, making us aware of the changes we needed to make in order to help support our parents and us as a family. Let's just say, my father has had a huge role in shaping the way I see the world and how it works.

He taught me how to read people's body language and express myself through the arts. He included me in collaboration on an award-winning American Red Cross theater performance program exploring community health issues such as AIDS/HIV, body image, and domestic violence. I also traveled to St. Louis with him as a teen to help with a gang violence prevention theater program. All along, I learned not only that the arts had the power to heal communities but also that providing this work required an entrepreneurial spirit.

After graduating from high school, I moved to Chicago to become a professional actor and study film directing at Columbia College Chicago. I booked several commercials, acted in a ton of plays, choreographed for and danced in music videos, and starred in a couple independent films. My big break came when I booked my first union job as a go-go dancer for a Wisconsin Lottery commercial. I loved performing. I loved directing. I wanted nothing more but to continue that love for the rest of my life.

When I was 21, my father passed away from a heart attack. I was lost for quite some time without his presence. I later stumbled upon an opportunity to do theater with inner city youth. They were some of the most troubled teens I had ever encountered, and they had little knowledge of the world's possibilities of growth due to their community's lack of safety and financial stability. Through theater, I saw these youth grow and learn about a world outside of their existence. They were able to give voice to their struggles and begin to form bonds not only with one another but also with the community.

After having worked with these youth in creating theater retellings of their life stories and bearing witness to tremendous change within these communities, both mentally and emotionally, I decided it was time to create a safe place for people to not only acquire mental health services, but also express themselves in creative ways. I also wanted to train other people on how to combine their love for the arts with their passion for healing others.

So, how did I do that? To be quite frank, I was faced with more "Nos" than "Yeses." It seemed as if everywhere I turned, people were telling me that I either wasn't capable of achieving this dream, or I didn't have the resources to do so. One thing people didn't know about me though, is that when I hear, "You can't," I work even harder to prove that "I can."

First Steps and Missteps

First things first. If I wanted to work with people struggling with mental health issues, I needed to know how to safely support them in their healing journey, so I began training at Kansas State University in their Alternative Drama Therapy Training program. The first time I stepped into a drama therapy classroom, I knew it was a place I could call home. I simultaneously began my master's program in Theatre, Communications, and Media at Northeastern Illinois University in Chicago.

While finishing up my graduate degree and drama therapy training, I was faced with an unforeseen challenge. In order to practice psychotherapy in the state of Illinois and be able to bill insurance as a private practitioner, I needed a mental health professional license. Enter stage two of training: I enrolled in the Community Counseling graduate program at Northeastern Illinois University in Chicago. Prior to entering this program, I felt as if I knew everything I needed to know about working in mental health. However, the supportive, yet challenging, counseling professors there taught me otherwise. I learned which theory of counseling worked best within the drama therapy framework. I harnessed my ability to read people's body language in a psychotherapeutic context. Most of all, I became a mental health professional who was now capable of using the arts in a safe and therapeutic way.

As for being able to train students to become a registered drama therapist (RDT), I spent the following five years practicing, directing, acting, and serving within my community as an RDT in order to become a board-certified trainer (BCT). My love for all of the arts also took me down the path of additional training in order to become a registered expressive arts therapist (REAT). I knew I didn't have enough time to become certified in all of the creative arts therapy professions, yet I wanted to make sure that I was inter-modally utilizing all of the arts for the benefit of my clients.

Now comes the hard part.

Taking the Leap into Entrepreneurship

I had no idea what I was doing when I decided to take the leap into entrepreneurship. Let me be crystal clear. No. Idea.

I started at the library. From accounting and marketing to writing business plans and business law, I immersed myself in every business book I could get my hands on. I learned how to file my business name with the state and federal jurisdictions, trademark my business name, set up an effective accounting management system, schedule my marketing and social media content, design a visually appealing search engine optimized website, design a welcoming office space, and secure a commercial real estate contract in a co-working office complex. This was just the preparation stage.

It was only after walking out of a job that no longer supported my dreams that I finally decided to put all of my preparation into action. My first step in getting people within the community to know about my new business was to reach out to every family medical practice in the area. If I was going to work primarily with children and teens, I needed to connect with the people who could refer potential clients for mental health services. I packed up my car with baskets of fresh-baked goods, my newly printed brochures and business cards, and a driver's seat full of possibilities, and started making the rounds. I made best friends with the receptionists, as the doctors were all inevitably busy, dropped off my basket of hopes and dreams, and simply let them know that I was in the area ready to support their patients. I followed up with a quick e-mail to each drop-off site to thank them for taking the time to talk with me. In came a couple referrals.

I also started to implement my marketing strategy for the training portion of my business by creating flyers, writing e-mail campaigns for people who signed up for my newsletter, visiting colleges and universities to talk about drama therapy as a career option for their students, and sharing resources with local mental health professionals looking to make a career change through social media. In came a couple more referrals.

After about year of this, I had built up a caseload of 15 clients, and the drama therapy training classes had, on average, six students. This sounds great, right? Nope. By this time, I had acquired a mountain of debt. I had charged up our family credit card to the max, my overhead was out of control due to the amount of money it was taking to get marketing materials printed, pay for the rental of an office space, utilities, website hosting, social media content platforms, parking for networking events, paid advertising in local magazines, and so on and so on.

If anyone tells you that opening up your own business is how you can make a ton of money, run the other way.

I started crying. What was I doing wrong? I thought I had read all the books and done everything I needed to do to run a successful business. Well, apparently, I hadn't. So, I finally made the decision to sit down with my partner, as he runs his own family-owned company and went over my numbers. Why was I in so much debt? How was I losing more money than I was making? Where was all the money going? More tears were shed. Pride was swallowed. Humility was restored. As my partner and I went through the year of profit and loss statements, I could see where money had been wasted (that huge and expensive ad with the local park district), and where money was being well spent (website hosting and search engine optimization). I learned exactly how to spend money in order to make an actual profit. I also made sure to examine my profit and loss statements each and every month to see what was working and not working within the financial aspects of my business. I started to see my business, the Center for Creative Arts Therapy, as an actual business. It was no longer just a dream. It was now a reality that I was responsible for seeing, not only survive, but flourish.

The contracts the Center for Creative Arts Therapies has with local organizations and schools have been instrumental in improving the emotional well-being and mental health of their faculty, staff, and students. One study we recently conducted with the Community Adult Day Center, a recreational, social, and intellectual program for adults who cannot safely be left alone, showed a 73% decrease in depression. Another contract in which we created an original musical with Trinity High School, an all-girl private high school, explored the personal stories of students and their experiences with bigotry, racism, alcoholism, along with their belief in a new day. Their participation in the creation and performance of their piece showed a 57% increase in self-esteem. After going through countless talk therapists, parents, who felt like no one could help their child, were able to decrease restrictions at home, saw an improvement in school behavior, and discovered their struggling child was better able to communicate their needs and express their emotions in a safe way.

Our training program has supported students who have gone on to use their knowledge in psychiatric hospitals in Trinidad, medical hospitals in Syria, orphanages in Africa, veteran treatment facilities in New York, theater organizations working with special needs children, and inner-city schools. By training the next generation of arts-based clinicians, our social impact has reached throughout the world, and we will continue to foster the next generation of pioneers.

The Center for Creative Arts Therapy is unique in that it is a one-stop shop for all of your arts-based psychotherapy and training needs. While there is currently one other organization in the state of Illinois offering arts-based psychotherapy, we are the only organization in the country that offers both arts-based psychotherapy services AND trains leading students toward both the registered drama therapist and registered expressive arts therapist credential. We are the only organization in the western suburbs of Chicago to offer all arts-based psychotherapy services for the community (art therapy, music therapy, dance/movement therapy, and drama therapy). We are also the only organization in the country that fosters a membership model for early childhood social-emotional learning, using the arts as its teaching modality.

Growth Pains

This all sounds great, right? Yes, it is. However, what I just shared about The Center for Creative Arts Therapy is simply the breakdown of accomplishments. It does not explore the many failures and challenges we have faced along the way.

As an entrepreneur, I get bored easily. I am constantly in creation mode, and sometimes I go down the rabbit hole of "new idea development" and forget to tend to the daily needs of my business. One such example was when I started a holistic, essential oils silly putty business. It failed due to the natural ingredients causing an unpleasant mold growth within the putty. The product was discontinued after six months of distribution.

Next was a class-based model in which people could come to take arts classes with our therapists and yoga instructors. We shelved this concept after confusion set in among our community about whether we were therapists or art teachers. There were a couple other ventures that led to the ultimate demise of an idea.

That being said, each and every failure taught me something that I now use to support my business. I learned how to implement membership models and reoccurring revenue streams of income. I learned how to secure patents, trademarks, and name registrations. I learned how to create product codes and design website content that spoke to different target audiences. I learned how to pivot strategies when they were no longer serving the needs of our business or community. I learned that natural ingredients cause mold when introduced to liquid. Most of all, I learned how to strategize.

My Advice

Perfection is the enemy of done. As I write this chapter, I am covered in a fine dust of insulation debris from construction going on at our house caused by a flood, chocolate syrup from my 7-year-old daughter's hands during a goodbye hug as she went off to a camping trip with my partner, and pen scribbles I wrote on my hand before bed, trying not to forget what I needed to do today. I have a "to do" list that goes on for three pages with additional "to dos" attached to the other "to dos."

Life as an entrepreneur is messy, literally and figuratively. You never know what will happen minute to minute, let alone what you may be covered in. Having a plan and then being able to deviate from that plan in order to push your business forward is important. You've got to roll with the punches, because if you wait to jump into your dreams at "just the right moment," that moment will never come. I have failed so many times trying to get things perfect, because perfection does not exist. It's just you and a dream, so go ahead and make it a reality.

MAGIC AS THERAPY!

▶ by Kevin Spencer

Kevin Spencer, MEd, specializes in the art of magic and illusion. He is faculty in the education department at Carlow University in Pittsburgh; a Fulbright specialist and a subject matter expert on arts integration for special populations for the US Department of State; a research consultant in the School of Health Professions, Department of Occupational Therapy and Institute of Arts in Medicine at the University of Alabama at Birmingham. He received the North American Performing Arts Agents and Managers (NAPAMA) Liz Silverstein Award for Agent-Manager of the Year. He has a master's in education, certification in autism studies, and is a PhD candidate in special education.

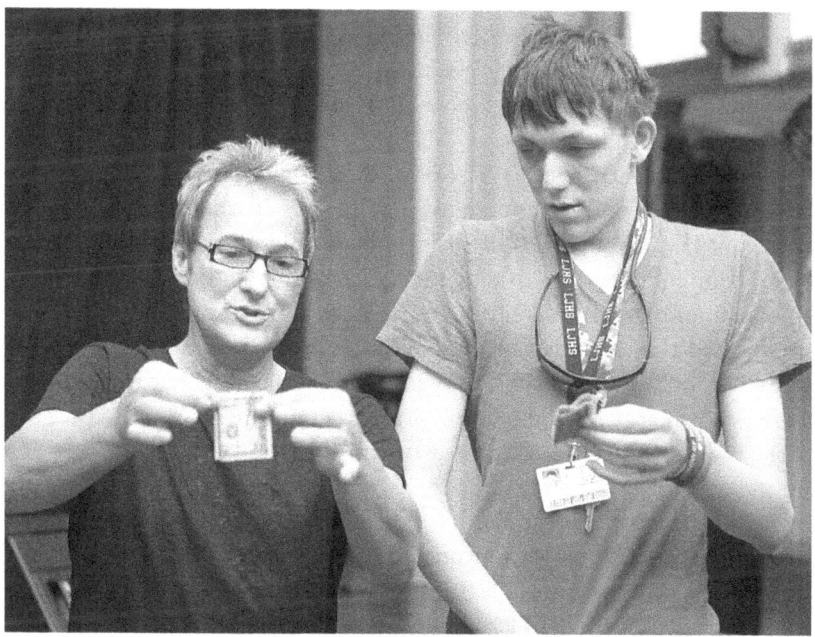

Figure 5.3 Kevin Spencer teaches the magic dollar bill trick to a student.

Beginnings

Performing magic tricks has been a part of my life for as long as I can remember. I saw my first magician perform on television when I was about 5-years-old, and I can remember telling my mom, "When I grow up, I'm going to be a magician!" My parents bought me a magic set for Christmas when I was eight and that was the beginning of a great adventure. I read magic books from the library and learned many tricks I could share with my friends. I carried them with me to elementary and middle school. Eventually, I worked my way through college doing magic shows. It was a natural transition from college to full-time performing, and I found my place in the world of entertainment rather quickly.

The Art of Magic

I'm fascinated by the art of magic. It has a story as old as recorded history. It may be the oldest and most universal of the performing arts because it easily translates from one culture to another. The Westcar Papyrus, dated 3500 BCE, records the performance of a magician in the Pharaoh's court. Cave paintings by prehistoric people in southern France and northern Spain contain images of magicians performing their tricks. Magicians performed in the streets and marketplaces of ancient Greece and Rome. And magicians of the past were an important part of society and significant players in the world of theater (Christopher & Christopher, 2005). Their problem-solving and creative abilities made significant contributions to modern civilization including the parachute, vending machines, pay toilets, and the technology used to show movies. They were often called the "scientists of show business" – daring, adventurous, and willing to attempt new impossibilities with no guarantee of success. In many ways, those who enter the world of creative arts therapy are magicians. They are some of the most effective and creative artists in the world.

I've long been a believer that the arts have the potential to make a difference in the realities in which we live, learn, work, and heal. Because of that conviction, I set out to investigate the impact learning and performing a few simple magic tricks might have on health and learning. Based on this research, I created two magic trick-based programs. The first is Magic Therapy™ which is used in a healthcare environment, often by occupational and speech therapists. The second program is called Hocus Focus™, and it was developed for use by teachers and therapists in schools for children with a special education classification and/or disability.

Those of us who work as magic performers know there is a process, a procedure for learning a new magic trick. My friend and mentor was a great magician named Doug Henning. He had a specific formula for learning magic that speaks loudly to those who work with individuals who have developmental and intellectual disabilities and those who have mental health concerns or have experienced trauma. Henning said, *"The difficult must become habit, habit becomes beautiful, and then beautiful becomes magic."*

When learning a new magic trick (or task), one practices the movements over and over again until they become muscle-memory or habitual – the ability to execute the moves without concentrating on sequencing the steps. Once this happens, one can begin to focus on ensuring that the movements are smooth and confident, performed with competence and finesse. With the first two steps of this formula complete, one can then present the magic trick (or task) to an "audience" for their enjoyment or approval.

Using Magic Tricks Therapeutically (Magic Therapy™)

The concept of using magic tricks therapeutically is the result of a volunteer experience one summer at a local hospital. My wife and I began teaching very basic, simple magic tricks to a small group of stroke patients. The therapists noticed significant improvement in some important areas of their recovery – cognition, motor skills, self-concept, and confidence. We started working with other patients in the hospital and then expanded into other rehab facilities teaching magic tricks to individuals with brain injuries, spinal cord injuries, and mental health diagnoses. We saw the same type of improvements with those individuals and began to explore further how magic tricks could be used therapeutically to motivate clients to become more engaged in their treatment program. Local and regional news stories brought the project to the attention of the American Medical Association, and the program was featured in the *Journal of the American Medical Association* (JAMA). This laid the foundation for what was to become a collaboration between a small group of therapists and my wife and I to develop a systematized, organized approach that would later become the Magic Therapy™ program. Today, the concepts of this project are supported by the American Occupational Therapy Association and are being effectively used in thousands of hospitals and rehabilitation centers in more than 30 countries.

The Model of Human Occupation provides a framework to understand the use of magic in this context. Central to this model are the interrelated components of volition, habituation, and performance capacity. Volition refers to the motivation to engage in the magic; habituation provides a process of organization of the magic into a routine; and performance capacity describes the physical and mental capacity required. All these dynamic components of a person are engaged through the "doing" of magic (Taylor, 2017). In addition, several theories play an underlying role in explaining learning to perform magic tricks as an effective intervention. The incentive theory of motivation (Killeen, 1982) supports the idea that learning to perform a magic trick may have a special appeal for individuals with a disability because it gives them a chance to do something that may not be replicated by their peers. Social learning theory (Bandura, 1977) corroborates the notion that people are often enthusiastic to practice magic tricks, even those that might be difficult, because performing for family and friends promotes socialization and personal growth.

The three stages detailed in motor learning theory (Zwicker & Harris, 2009) are especially relevant to the process of learning to perform a magic trick. During the first stage (cognitive), the client may have a general understanding of the movements required to perform the trick but might not be certain how to execute those movements. The second stage is an explicit learning stage (associative). As a result of regular practice, the execution of the movements becomes more refined and performed with greater consistency. The client's focus is on attaining the goal of mastering the magic trick, requiring less guidance, and consciously adapting and adjusting movements independently (Muratori, Lamberg, Quinn, & Duff, 2013). In the final stage (autonomous), the client has learned the motor skills and requires little cognitive effort to perform the trick.

Research Findings

The therapeutic use of magic tricks is supported by robust scientific research. Incorporating magic tricks in therapy can serve to motivate clients to practice outside of regular therapy sessions (Green et al., 2013; Hines, Bundy, Black, Haertsch, & Wallen, 2019). Fieldwork on magic trick integration and traumatic brain injury won first poster prize at the Canadian Association of Physical Medicine and Rehabilitation Meeting in Toronto (Kwong & Cullen, 2007). Research using magic tricks as an intervention with mental health diagnoses won first poster prize at the International Mental Health Conference in Hong Kong (Sui & Sui, 2007). Research on using magic tricks as a themed approach to hand-arm bimanual intensive therapy for children with hemiplegia won first poster prize at the European Academy of Childhood Disabilities Conference (Green et al., 2013), and further studies have demonstrated significant results with this population (Green et al., 2013; Hines et al., 2019; Schertz et al., 2016;

Spencer et al., 2020, Weinstein et al., 2015). I believe in the effectiveness of using magic tricks in rehabilitation because the art of illusion has the ability to capture and hold the attention of people of all ages. Everyone is intrigued by the seeming impossibility of a magic trick.

Magic can help improve skills like communication and socialization, because magic tricks are meant to be performed for an audience. Much like storytelling, magic allows the person performing the trick to create his/her own narrative. Magic taps into the cognitive processes: the planning and sequence of steps. Magic tricks are effective in increasing a client's ability to manipulate objects (fine motor dexterity), as well as gross motor skills: magic allows mastery of the environment without requiring skillful hand movements. The repetitive action of practicing a magic trick can help build up strength and dexterity and, consequently, help to increase independence. The performance skills taught as part of the magic learning experience are used to increase the participants' communication skills, confidence, self-esteem, and emotional well-being. Magic provides cognitive and perceptual challenges and can be used to increase frustration tolerance, task follow-through, concentration, cooperation, and impulse control. Magic may have a significant impact on neurodevelopmental functions, such as neuro-motor, attention, memory, language, temporal-sequential ordering, spatial ordering, social cognition, and other higher order cognition. The learning and performing of magic tricks can allow individuals to safely explore their skill level while providing a fun way of reaching therapeutic goals, regardless of age, ability, or function.

When occupational therapists use magic tricks to engage their clients in therapy, they no longer need to use dated and mundane therapeutic tasks. Instead, learning magic tricks provides a fun and motivating way to develop the necessary skills required to perform the trick for others. Because of the level of engagement, it is often an occupation that clients will continue outside of therapy. They will carry it home and continue to improve, taking every opportunity to show their friends and family the skills they have acquired, exhibiting a sense of pride and belonging. At the same time, they reach their therapeutic goals, often without even being aware of it. A carefully selected series of tricks achieves these goals while the client merely thinks they are learning and performing "magic."

Magic Tricks in the Classroom (Hocus Focus™)

Based on the success and results of the research in the medical field, I was confident there was a way that magic tricks could be used to help students

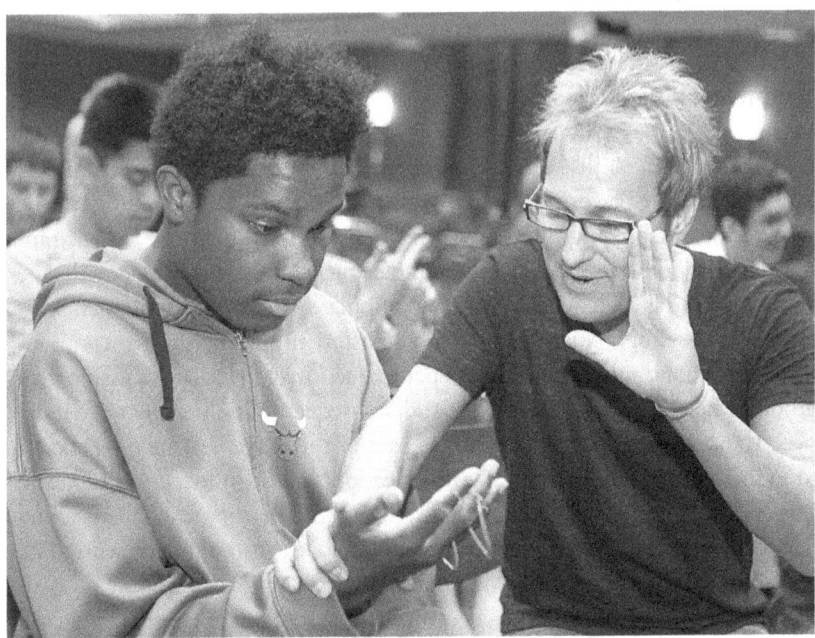

Figure 5.4 Kevin Spencer teaches magic to a student.

with disabilities improve the skills they find challenging. In the late 20th century, a small number of education researchers evaluated the effectiveness of using magic tricks with students who had a classified learning disability. The results revealed that: (1) magic tricks offer a creative means for stimulating the senses in special education students (Frith & Walker, 1983); (2) magic tricks enhance the learning experience and encourage creative problem-solving skills, observational techniques, and critical thinking (McCormack, 1985); (3) magic tricks provide a strategy for building teamwork and self-esteem in children with Emotional Behavior Disorder (Broome, 1989); and (4) teaching magic tricks in an educational setting can help students with learning differences attain higher self-esteem and self-confidence (Ezell & Ezell, 2003).

While these studies showed positive results, there was no further research for several years. More recent research has shown that using a magic trick-based curriculum in which academics and functional skills are embedded into learning and performance encourages students to create a context and communicate that through movement and storytelling (Spencer, 2012; Spencer & Balmer, 2020). Our students need to develop their creativity, critical thinking, and problem-solving skills, but they also need to be able to communicate effectively, collaborate with people different from themselves, demonstrate initiative, and be self-directed. One of the biggest challenges for educators is finding activities that are engaging and meaningful for their students. Even more challenging is finding activities that allow for inter-disciplinary collaborations between educators, speech language pathologists, psychologists, counselors, and occupational therapists to help our children achieve their desired outcomes. That is the focus of the Hocus Focus™ program.

Several studies have concluded that using magic tricks to deliver academic and functional content to children and adolescents with a variety of disability classifications, including autism and emotional disturbance, can allow them to experience academic successes as well as change the way they believe others perceive them, helping them with social acceptance. Learning magic has a special appeal for children, because it gives them a chance to do something that can't be equaled by their peers. This can promote socialization and personal growth.

Humans are designed to seek social relationships with an emphasis on belonging, being recognized, listened to, and noticed. Research supports the idea that learning is most effective when it is social and collaborative. By integrating magic tricks into the education process, students can engage in purposeful conversation. And they depend on each other's thinking to enrich their understanding and construct meaning. This cooperative learning process is a valuable experience for children. Helping one another stirs creativity and builds positive relationships. It also increases a student's feeling of control over his environment and improves self-esteem. This can be a transformative experience for a child or adolescent who struggles.

CPR Analytics is a validated assessment instrument that allows teachers and therapists to measure student outcomes in five domains – cognition, motor skills, communication, social skills, and flexible thinking – using an arts-based approach (O'Rourke, Spencer, & Kelly, 2018).

Magic Tricks and Creative Arts Therapies

For decades, professionals who are actively engaged in working with those who have disabilities or mental health concerns have recognized the benefits of an arts integrated approach, one that engages the whole person and allows for alternative ways of receptive and expressive communication and avoids the limitations of language. Enhancing communication is a critical component of the healing process, and the arts open opportunities for improved therapeutic outcomes. The arts may provide a window for clients to reveal underlying emotions. We recognize that giving our clients the right set of circumstances and creating a safe environment encourages the expression of feelings, thoughts, and ideas which may be beneficial in solving conflicts, managing behaviors, improving self-esteem, developing self-awareness and insight, managing stress, and developing interpersonal skills.

Many art disciplines bring with them an assumption of competence; that is, there is an expectation that we might know how to sing a song, move our bodies to music, or draw a picture of a person, object, or event. But an important consideration of creative arts therapies is that clients are not required to have any artistic skills. The only prerequisite is their willingness to engage their imagination, feeling, and awareness to process and support their healing. One of the advantages of learning and performing magic is there are no pre-conceived expectations of their knowledge or ability to perform a trick. Who (but a trained magician) should know how to do a magic trick? This understanding gives them permission to take risks and make mistakes. Learning something new – like a magic trick – brings with it the realization that one will make a mistake. And mistakes are not only expected, they are accepted. When we allow children and adolescents to be creative, we remove the stressors of being right and through their mistakes, they develop important skills like resilience, flexibility, adaptability, critical thinking, and problem-solving.

Research confirms that curiosity triggers motivation, and motivation is a critical component for success (Fell, 2014). The attraction of learning a magic trick may increase the motivation of an individual to engage in their treatment program. While we saw significant improvements in many areas in our research, building a positive self-concept, self-confidence, and self-efficacy were crucial elements to the success of our clients (Spencer, 2012; Spencer & Balmer, 2020; Spencer, Yuen, Jenkins, Kirklin Griffin, Vogtle, & Davis, 2020).

Magic Therapy™ and Trauma

Performing a magic trick requires more than the ability to simply sequence and execute the moves. The performer must also be able to engage the audience through the telling of a story (patter) and the use of appropriate gestures to highlight the impossibility of the presentation. It also requires an understanding of the "secret move," the specific steps or actions that must be hidden from the audience for the magic to work. The performer completes a series of movements which are obvious and visible to them; but the audience sees something completely different – an impossibility, a magical phenomenon! This distinction can be used to demonstrate that people see things from different perspectives and, often, what they see can be very different.

The selection of magic tricks for a client can also have an impact on their success and, consequently, on their therapeutic progress. Carefully selecting tricks that allow for immediate success and gratification in the first few sessions will encourage them to work harder as the tricks become more difficult and complex. And with the mastery of these more challenging tricks, they become more confident in their abilities. But there are other outcomes that are equally as beneficial – the client's awareness of their own thinking, understanding, and knowledge. When our clients develop knowledge about how they learn and then gain the potential to apply this knowledge, they become more effectively equipped to apply what they've learned to solve problems.

The Concepts of SIAM

Several years ago, I created this acronym to help me remember the distinct attributes that the creative arts therapies, including the use of magic tricks, bring to the healing process: self-expression, imagination, active participation, and mind-body connections. Each of these areas can help people by strengthening resilience through social supports, developing a positive view of oneself, realizing that change is possible, and keeping things in perspective.

Self-expression

All effective therapies encourage clients to engage in self-exploration and expression. Research suggests that the use of the arts in psychotherapy may accelerate this process and encourage a deeper self-understanding that may result in a sense of well-being and a resolution of conflict (Gladding, 1992). For those who have suffered a traumatic experience, thoughts and feelings are not exclusively stored in the brain as verbal language. The use of creative approaches can offer an important way of helping these individuals discover and communicate memories, feelings, and thoughts. Learning a magic trick brings together multiple skills and abilities and encourages self-expression in the performance.

Imagination

Imagination is the wonderful ability to conjure images and ideas in our mind without any immediate input to our other senses. It is an essential component of creativity, problem-solving, and self-expression. The creative arts therapies focus on the process of creating rather than the artistic outcome. This process engages the client's imaginative thinking and uses their senses, giving rise to self-expression and discovery that may lead to resolution and reparation.

Performing a magic trick allows individuals to take on a different identity (the magician), performing as someone other than themselves. In the safety of this character, they often share their fears, hopes, and desires through the story they tell when performing their magic trick.

Active participation

All therapies require clients to participate in the process. Psychology defines creative arts therapies as action therapies (Weiner, 1999). These methods and techniques go beyond merely asking clients to participate. They require clients to become fully involved, to invest themselves in the process, redirecting their awareness to visual, tactile, and auditory channels. Magic Malchiodi (2005) writes, "The experience of doing, making, and creating actually energizes individuals, redirects attention and focus, and alleviates emotional stress, allowing clients to fully concentrate on issues, goals, and behaviors" (p. 10). Performing a magic trick necessitates the active participation of clients – mind and body.

Mind-body connection

The mind-body connection is not a new approach in healthcare, but the 20th century did bring new investigations that scientifically demonstrate the complex relationship between the mind and body. Research is discovering that thoughts, emotions, beliefs, and attitudes contribute to chemical imbalances in the body. Our thoughts, feelings, and attitudes can negatively or positively affect our biological functioning.

Understanding this holistic approach is characteristic of the creative arts therapies. Practitioners capitalize on the sensory aspects of engaging in the process of making art, but they also empower people to recognize their natural abilities and skills, both of which can bring about change in the life of a client.

For more information:

Magic Therapy™ – MagicTherapy.com
Hocus Focus™ – HocusFocusEducation.com

References

Bandura, A. (1977). *Social learning theory*. Prentice-Hall.

Broome, S. A. (1989). *The Magic Kids: A strategy to build self-esteem and change attitudes toward the handicapped*. Paper presented at the 67th annual convention of the Council for Exceptional Children. San Francisco, CA.

Christopher, M., & Christopher, M. (2005). *The illustrated history of magic*. Carroll & Graf Publishers.

Ezell, D., & Ezell, C. (2003). M.A.G.I.C.W.O.R.K.S. (Motivating activities geared to instilling confidence wonderful opportunities to raise kid's self-esteem). *Education and Training in Developmental Disabilities, 30*(4), 441–450.

Fell, A. (2014, October 2). Curiosity helps learning and memory. [Weblog comment]. Retrieved from http://blogs.ucdavis.edu/egghead/2014/10/02/curiosity-helps-learning-and-memory/

Frith, G. H., & Walker, J. C. (1983). Magic as motivation for handicapped students. *Teaching Exceptional Children, 15*(2), 108–110.

Gladding, S. (1992). *Counseling as an art: The creative arts in counseling*. American Counseling Association.

Green, D., Schertz, M., Gordon, A. M., Moore, A., Schejter Margalit, T., Farquharson, Y., ... Fattal-Valevski, A. (2013). A multi-site study of functional outcomes following a themed approach to hand-arm bimanual intensive therapy for children with hemiplegia. *Developmental Medicine & Child Neurology, 55*(6), 527–533. doi:10.1111/dmcn.12113

Hines, A., Bundy, A. C., Black, D., Haertsch, M., & Wallen, M. (2019). Upper limb function of children with unilateral cerebral palsy after a magic-themed HABIT: A pre-post- study with 3- and 6-month follow-up. *Physical & Occupational Therapy in Pediatrics, 39*(4), 404–419. doi:10.1080/01942638.2018.1505802

Killeen, P. R. (1982). Incentive theory: II. Models for choice. *Journal of the Experimental Analysis of Behavior, 38*(2), 217–232. doi:10.1901/jeab.1982.38-217

Kwong, E. H., & Cullen, N. (2007, June 13–16) *Do you believe in magic? Teaching magic to patients as an adjunct to their rehabilitation program*. Canadian Association of Physical Medicine and Rehabilitation Annual Meeting, London, ON (poster presentation).

Malchiodi, C. A. (Ed.). (2005). *Expressive therapies*. The Guilford Press.

McCormack, A. J. (1985). Teaching with magic: Easy ways to hook your class on science. *Learning, 14*(1), 62–67.

Muratori, L. M., Lamberg, E. M., Quinn, L., & Duff, S. V. (2013). Applying principles of motor learning and control to upper extremity rehabilitation. *Journal of Hand Therapy, 26*(2), 94–102. quiz 103. doi:10.1016/j.jht.2012.12.007

O'Rourke, S., Spencer, K., & Kelly, F. (2018). Development and psychometric investigation of an arts integrated assessment instrument for educators. *Journal for Learning Through the Arts, 14*(1). Retrieved from https://escholarship.org/uc/item/0mx5z5xd, doi: 10.21977/D914137309

Schertz, M., Shiran, S. I., Myers, V., Weinstein, M., Fattal-Valevski, A., Artzi, M., ... Green, D. (2016). Imaging predictors of improvement from a motor learning-based intervention for children with unilateral cerebral palsy. *Neurorehabilitation and Neural Repair, 30*(7), 647–660. doi:10.1177/1545968315613446

Spencer, K., & Balmer, S. (2020). A pilot study: Magic tricks in the ELL classroom increasing verbal communication initiative and self-efficacy. *English Language Teaching and Linguistics Studies, 2*(1), 11-32. doi:10.22158/eltls.v2n1p11

Spencer, K. (July 2012). Hocus Focus: Evaluating the benefits of magic tricks with special populations. *Journal of the International Association of Special Education, 13*(1), 87–99.

Spencer, K., Yuen, H., Jenkins, G. Kirklin, K., Griffin, A. Vogtle, L., & Davis, D. (2020). Evaluation of a magic camp for children with hemiparesis: A pilot study. *Occupational Therapy in Health Care, 34*(2), 155-170. doi:10.1080/07380577.2020.1741055

Sui, P., & Sui, M. (2007, December). *Use of magic: Creative means for psychosocial rehabilitation*. Presentation at International Health and Mental Health Conference Hong Kong.

Taylor, R. (2017). *Kielhofner's model of human occupation: Theory and application.* Wolters Kluwer.

Weiner, D. (1999). *Beyond talk therapy: Using movement and expressive techniques in clinical practice.* American Psychological Association. doi:10.1037/10326-000.

Weinstein, M., Myers, V., Green, D., Schertz, M., Shiran, S. I., Geva, R., ... Ben Bashat, D. (2015). Brain plasticity following intensive bimanual therapy in children with hemiparesis: Preliminary evidence. *Neural Plasticity,* 2015, 1–13. doi:10.1155/2015/798481

Zwicker, J. G., & Harris, S. R. (2009). A reflection on motor learning theory in pediatric occupational therapy practice. *Canadian Journal of Occupational Therapy, 76*(1), 29–37. doi:10.1177/000841740907600108

BECOMING ADVOCATES FOR OUR CLIENTS AND OUR FIELDS

▶ A Conversation With Michelle Yadon and Tracena Marie

Michelle Yadon, MA, CTRS, RDT-BCT, CPRP is a registered drama therapist in Carmel, Indiana who has worked for the Stone Belt ARC and currently is the recreation manager of programming for the Carmel Clay Parks and Recreation Department. She received the 2019 NADTA Performance Award.

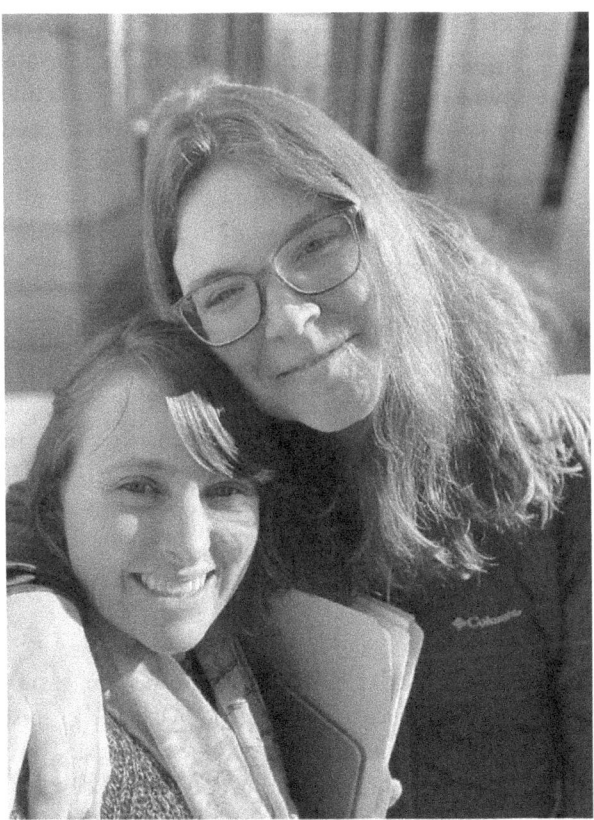

Figure 5.5 Drama therapists Tracena Marie (left) and Michelle Yadon (right).

Tracena Marie, MA, RDT, is a registered drama therapist in Muncie, Indiana who directs a Barrier-Free Theatre program for Muncie Civic Theatre, has a private practice, and is an adjunct instructor of theater at Ball State University.

MICHELLE: I went to school for drama therapy because I wanted to learn how to utilize drama therapy with people with disabilities. I always wanted to work in a community center, which I do now. I think it's very important to work on systemic issues within a community, building the community's strengths and supporting the individuals in it.

TRACENA: I'm Tracena Marie, and I live in Muncie, Indiana. Currently, the majority of my work includes group therapy contracts affiliated with organizations in my community. I facilitate a Barrier-Free Theatre program at my local community theater and teach an introduction to drama therapy course for undergraduate students at Ball State University. After graduating from Northwestern State University of Louisiana with my bachelor's degree in Theatre, I knew I wanted to utilize theater in a way that could serve and empower others. I began to research the different ways to incorporate my theater background and training. Drama therapy came up in my search, and I thought, "This sounds really cool, I should look into this because I can see myself doing this work." So, I did, and I became fascinated with the field of drama therapy, and I knew I wanted to be a part of this profession. I've met so many wonderful people in the drama therapy community who have really helped me get to where I am now, and I just want to acknowledge that because I do believe that this community is founded on supporting each other.

MICHELLE: Tracena and I were the first two drama therapists in Indiana. I lived in Indianapolis, which is about 45 minutes from Muncie, so we started to come together, have lunches, and brainstorm. If we couldn't have lunches, we would talk on the phone. We said, "We're the first two drama therapists in Indiana, so how do we want drama therapy to be developed in the state? We get to decide." We wrote our ideas down. One of the things we wanted to do was bring more drama therapists into the state. Tracena was the one who had the idea to get on the state Medicaid waiver as a way to fund our services for our clients who don't make a lot of money.

The Medicaid waiver is a provision in the Medicaid law that allows certain regulations to be "waived" in order to provide payment for services for Medicaid clients. Waivers are different in every state, and there are different processes involved. There are different types of waivers: ones for people who have intellectual and developmental disabilities (IDD), for older adults, for mental health services. The waiver that Tracena and I focused on was the one for people with IDD. In Indiana there are two different kinds of waivers for people with IDD: the family-based waiver and the community-support waiver. The state wanted to keep people out of institutions. The family waiver was developed in 2010 so people could get services when they lived with their families. The community support waiver is for people living in a group home or apartment on their own. On the waivers there are different services that you can utilize: respite care, therapy, employment, mental health, and education. People work with a case manager and get this money for these services. Currently under the therapy section, recreational therapy and music therapy are listed as fundable services.

TRACENA: I believe there were nine music therapists living in the state when music therapy was written into the waiver service. This new line of funding meant there were new jobs for music therapists. Currently, there are over 300 music therapists working in the state under the waiver, and there's even a wait list for services because there aren't enough music therapists (or recreational therapists) to meet the demand of individuals on the waiver.

MICHELLE: Once Tracena heard about the waiver, we decided to make a list of 12 different people and organizations that we needed to talk to in order to find out more. We split them up between ourselves, and we started calling people, knocking on doors, having lunch with people. We talked to music therapists, we talked to rec therapists, we talked to different organizations that work with clients who have a stake getting services from the waiver.

TRACENA: It's important to find people who have a similar mission statement or, as Nancy Sondag would say, your "Why."[1] That is what's been driving Michelle and me. We believe in the mission of providing drama therapy to as many clients as possible, because we know how effective it is for them. So, being able to connect with other professionals who believe in the same type of mission or have the same philosophy has really made that process a little bit less daunting, more inviting. When I call people and talk to them or e-mail them, I know that what they are doing is something very similar to our mission as therapists.

MICHELLE: Once we started to get people on board, we started thinking of our quest to be part of the waiver as a business. We had a mission, developed a website, business cards, and a gmail account that we still use: rdtindiana@gmail.com.

In late 2017, we set up a meeting with the director of disabilities and rehabilitation services (DDRS) for the state of Indiana who administers this waiver. We

---

1 Your "WHY" is your purpose, your cause, your belief in *why* you do what you do. Your "WHY" drives your vision and your actions. It's not enough to say what you do and how you are different, you need to explain *why* you do it and find others who believe what you believe or convert them to believe in what you believe. The "WHY" concept of selling was codified by Simon Sinek in his book *Start with the Why*.

called and said, "Hello, this is who we are, we know that music therapy and recreational therapy are on the waiver, we'd like to set up a meeting with you, when can we meet?" A lot of professionals are required to take 24 – 48 hours to get back to you – that's their departmental policy. A lot of people will at least set up a meeting with you. She had her assistant contact us and set up a meeting. Then we started researching her.

TRACENA: Yes, let's just say we did quite a bit of research into the director's position and what that meant in relation to Medicaid waiver services. It's important to know your audience when proposing a new idea. Who are you telling your story to? What do they believe in? So, we learned that she had her own personal experiences with her brother living with a disability, and her role as a mother contributed to her accepting the position as the director of DDRS. I think being curious about her and the work she does made a big difference. This helped us approach our meeting in a more personal way.

MICHELLE: And then we went in for the meeting. We made a packet of materials: brochures, research articles, facts and figures. We explained drama therapy and the similarities and differences it has to talk therapy and the other creative arts therapies. We talked about our clients and how we saw drama therapy impacting their lives.

TRACENA: We started with a narrative story. That's what Michelle and I do best. We come from a theater background, and we understand the power or impact that our individual stories have, but also the story of the collective. Instead of handing her a bunch of research and numbers (which we still did, of course), we needed her to first understand the positive impact that drama therapy can have on a person. We opened our meeting with Michelle sharing a narrative case study about a person she works with at Carmel Clay Parks and Recreation. I think that allowed the DDRS director in the meeting to visualize our work because it was through a personal story. We had questions prepared, too. I think our questions allowed us to have an engaging conversation, and it provided us with insight and ideas, too, for how to move forward onto the next phase.

MICHELLE: At that meeting, the DDRS director let us know that the waiver was going to be redesigned in 2019. Whenever that happens things can be added to the waiver, changed, or taken away. She let us know that it would be very important to get support from parents and from key organizations that support people with disabilities.

TRACENA: We shared with her that if drama therapy is on the waiver, it would alleviate some of the overloaded caseloads that the music therapists have, as we are creative arts therapists who have equivalent education and similar training.

MICHELLE: She actually gave us the names of the people who it would be important to talk to about drama therapy, so we split up who we were going to contact and started having lunch and talking about why we wanted to be on the waiver. Simultaneously, we drafted a letter that we sent to parents of our clients and also different stakeholders that we wanted to send letters to the DDRS director and the waiver committee. It seemed to us, the more people who could hear the words "drama therapy," the more likely we could get on the waiver. We started doing free workshops and really pushed to get our work on the news, which we did several times. Every time we had a Playback Theatre show or a Barrier-Free show, we would send out tickets and flyers and invitations to people who needed to be in the know. Tracena insisted that we write out the invitations, not just send them a flyer. When they came to our shows, we would always point out to the audience that someone from this important organization was there, and that it was a really big deal.

TRACENA: One component to help us explain drama therapy has been the free workshops we've offered for organizations. Sometimes I find when we talk about drama therapy, it can be hard for people to grasp what it is, to visualize it. It's almost like they need to see it or experience it. Offering workshops for an organization's clients or staff members has been very successful. And usually, they ask me back or want to see more. It's a great way to market myself. I've learned how to ask, "Can I leave my brochure or my flyer or business card?" This past summer, I contacted a summer camp director and said, "Can I come lead a drama group for free and pass out my brochures?" I gained a child client that I work with out of that free workshop. It's been a bit of trial and error in thinking outside the box. Anytime you step outside your own door, looking for that connection can feel scary, but you need to do it because there might be someone out there who is willing to connect.

MICHELLE: During this time, I started supervising other creative arts therapists. I was supervising a dance/movement therapy student. Now there are three registered dance/movement therapists in Indiana, but a year ago there was only one. I wanted to make sure my student was taken care of, so we also started advocating for all of the creative arts therapies to get on the waiver. We started taking literature about all the different creative arts therapies with us, and we met with the art therapists and dance/movement therapists. We plan on having a weekend workshop with all of the creative arts therapists in our state in the next year and starting a listserve. We've started advocating for all the creative arts therapies to get on the waiver for folks with disabilities.

We send the director of DDRS an e-mail every three or four months, "Hey, remember us? We're the drama therapists you talked to!" "Hey, look at this article on the creative arts!" "Hey, we're having another play! We'd love for you to come!"

She strongly suggested that we attend task force meetings. Once a month the task force would meet in a different part of the state, and she made it very clear to us that it was important for us to go to those task force meetings and just say anything about drama therapy.

TRACENA: The task force meetings are still taking place – right now there are even more of them because we are closer to the end of this phase in the process. For anyone interested in learning about your own state's Medicaid waiver services, you can go on your state government's official website and should be able to find available task force meetings for waiver services. At these meetings, you can sometimes provide public comments. I've found that every meeting we have attended has been very informative and educational. We've met other professionals like case workers and recreational therapists who we otherwise would not have met. We request their contact information and put them on our e-mail list to keep them informed about drama therapy updates in our state.

MICHELLE: Tracena and I really support each other, and we are really honest about what we need, so we can help each other. Like sometimes I will start using jargon or sometimes my words will be confusing, so Tracena jumps in and explains. When Tracena felt nervous about talking at first, I would talk, and vice versa. We always hold the space for each other and support each other. We know each other's strengths, and we play off each other really well.

TRACENA: At the beginning it was very scary for me. There were unspoken questions I had like, "Were we worthy enough?" "Are we doing the right thing?" Second guessing ourselves. But our conversation with the DDRS director took away a lot of that fear. The whole goal started to become more tangible, something we could latch on to. She came across as another human being rather than her being this big entity.

MICHELLE: Where we are today: In January 2020, another task force meeting was organized, at which the committee was going to talk about the waiver redesign. The committee gave all of their ideas to an organization that they were contracting out to form the literature for the waiver. We got to the meeting, and they announced they were going to restructure the waivers, so instead of being two waivers, there will be three. They talked about all the new things they were going to put in – and there it was up on the screen, "expressive therapies." It included us! We were among all these "suits," and my lips started to quiver, and my eyes teared up.

That's where we are today. Now they are asking for public comments. They want to get families and other organizations to write in and say what they like about the new waiver and what they don't like about it. That's why we sent a letter out to all the drama therapists, organizations, people who helped us, our participants, and we told them what to say. All the state needs to know is that people want drama therapy to be on the waiver. They want to see the word drama therapy over and over again.

TRACENA: It's looking like the new waivers will be implemented early in 2022, so we still have a little way to go.

MICHELLE: Once we get on the waiver, we're not done. The next project is licensure, but we thought if we got on the waiver that would help us get licensure. I don't think this is necessary for every situation, but we thought it would be good in our state. We are hoping that by increasing communication between creative arts therapists in the state that we can come together and work together for licensure. We really want creative arts therapists from all the modalities in our state to be supportive of each other. In our meetings, a few of our creative arts colleagues told us that they tried to get licensure passed a number of years ago, but they couldn't get it through. We feel it may be important to show that creative arts therapists are waiver providers in order to be taken seriously by the legislature.

TRACENA: We also want to see drama therapy reach the other waivers. I, for one, would love for drama therapy to be on the waiver for older adults.

MICHELLE: And now we have more drama therapists in the state, so there will be lots of work for everyone.

TRACENA: It's been quite a few years – it's gone by fast. It's been very challenging, but I have never felt alone in this process. I think for us the biggest thing was who to connect with and finding our friends in our community. A big part of that was connecting with the therapists who were already on the waiver.

ONCE UPON A DREAM

▶ by Mizuho Kanazawa and
Barbara McKechnie

Mizuho Kanazawa, MA, LPC, LCAT, RDT–BCT, is a Japanese drama therapist in private practice in New York and New Jersey, serving clients who feel they are "between cultures." Her website can be found at www.dramaforhealing.com

Barbara McKechnie, MA, LPC, LCAT, RDT–BCT, TEP, is a drama therapist and psychodramatist who has worked with children, adolescents, and adults in both inpatient and partial hospital settings. She is past president of NADTA and NJACC and is a faculty member at Montclair State University in New Jersey. She currently works as a consultant, psychodrama trainer, and in private practice in NJ.

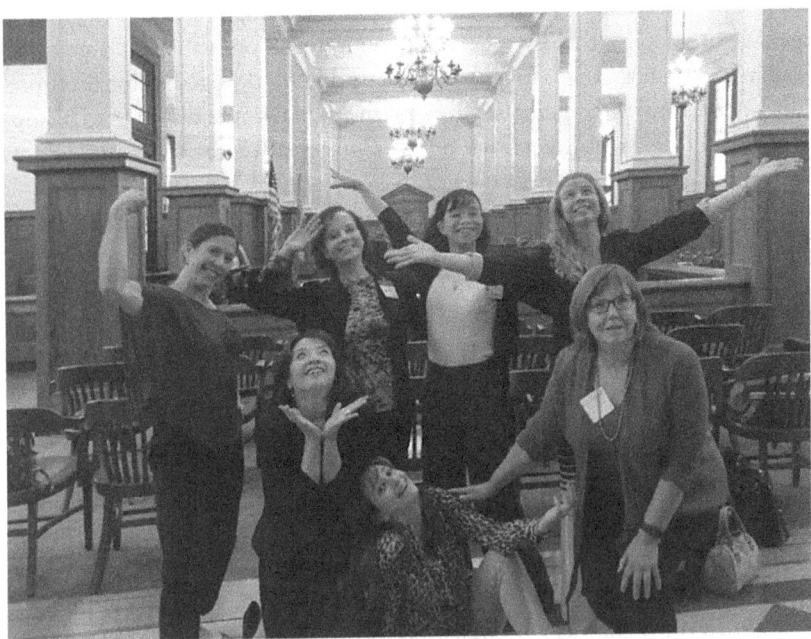

Figure 5.6 Members of the New Jersey Task Force for Licensure of Drama Therapists and Dance/Movement Therapists, Trenton, NJ: (l. to r.) Kristin Pollock, Mizuho Kanazawa, Tina Erfer, LisaGail Schwartz, Eri Millrod, Brooke Campbell, and Barbara McKechnie, September 26, 2016.

Once upon a time in the far away land of New Jersey, in the year of 2013, there was a drama therapist who wanted to be licensed in the state where she lived and worked. She heard that *art therapists* had a bill pending for licensure. She felt empowered to think more concretely about the possibility of licensure for *drama therapists*. She initially reached out to her drama therapist colleagues, and they agreed that *all* creative arts therapists should be licensed, and the collaboration can give them more power. So, they contacted dance/movement therapists and formed a team of dedicated professionals who became the NJ Task Force for Licensure of Drama Therapists and Dance/Movement Therapists.

Why is it important to license these professions? Drama therapy and dance/movement therapy are behavioral health disciplines that integrate psycho-therapeutic principles with theater, dance/movement, and the creative process. Fundamental mental health, psychological, developmental, and mind-body principles are utilized to support the emotional, physical, cognitive, and social well-being of individuals, families, and groups across the lifespan.

We, drama therapists and dance/movement therapists, work with those who are often the most vulnerable populations, including but not limited to veterans; those with Alzheimer's disease; developmental disabilities; severe and persistent mental illness; or autism; and those who suffer from domestic violence, child abuse, or substance abuse. We felt that a New Jersey state license would protect these individuals from possible harm by unlicensed and untrained practitioners.

As performing artists, when we start a production, we begin with an empty stage. We have no cast, no script, no props, no sets, no audience. We just have an idea and a dream. Starting the journey to licensure was like having an empty stage. It felt daunting, and we had no idea where we were going. We simply learned and found out one step at a time. Legislators who saw our actions and efforts began responding to our requests and need for support when they saw our seriousness and commitment to this dream.

Many New Jersey Creative Arts Therapists were licensed to work in New York as Licensed Creative Arts Therapists (LCAT) but not in the state where they resided. In 2006, Creative Arts Therapists were able to be licensed as Licensed Professional Counselors (LPC) in NJ during a brief period when the license for counselors first took effect. In order to obtain this expedited license, it was necessary to show that one met the criteria of training, education, and experience expected of a Licensed Professional Counselor. However, at the time of the formation of the NJ Task Force for Licensure of Drama Therapists and Dance/

Movement Therapists, this opportunity was no longer available to other creative arts therapists as the period of expedition had been closed for many years.

Because creative arts therapists have been able to demonstrate that their training was equivalent to other state licensed professionals, it seemed arbitrary, if not unethical, for them not to have access to the licensure process. Seeing that the art therapy bill was pending at this time, the thought of licensure for drama therapy and dance/movement therapy seemed more possible, so the journey began.

Establishing a hard-working, focused, passionate, and dedicated team was the easy part. Moving our licensure bill forward, step by step, became a rollercoaster of highs and lows, of successes and failures. Time seems to move very slowly in the legislative process! And having any control over what happens is often just an illusion.

Our process began with meetings with Assembly sponsors and the writing of the bill itself, which went through several versions. We made a conscious effort to make our bill comparable to the already established Professional Counselor bill and the pending Art Therapy bill. The path to becoming a drama therapist or dance/movement therapist is to earn a master's degree in Drama Therapy or in Dance/Movement Therapy (see Chapter 2 for descriptions of these processes). Great consideration was made to be inclusive of those drama therapists and dance/movement therapists who had trained as alternative track students. The alternate track drama therapy training and the alternative track dance/movement therapy training involves obtaining a master's degree in a mental health discipline, such as social work, psychology, or counseling and additional specific training in either drama therapy or dance/movement therapy. New Jersey licensure will apply to professionals who graduated from master's programs in drama therapy and dance/movement therapy as well as the alternative track trained drama therapists and dance/movement therapists.

There was the excitement of having legislators really listen to what we had to say and express support for our bill. We left those meetings feeling elated. However, each meeting left us with more questions than answers. We found out what we needed to do in each step of the process.

Each task force member reached out to their assembly legislators and senators to ask them to become the sponsors and cosponsors of our bill. We asked our families and colleagues to write to their representatives. We also reached out to drama therapists and dance/movement therapists within and outside of the state. We reached out to the North American Drama Therapy Association and American Dance Therapy Association for support. We arranged to have a special meeting inviting drama therapists and dance/movement therapists to learn about licensure and advocacy. In this process, we wanted to gauge, to make sure that licensure is a process that had the support of the whole community from NJ as well as from national organizations.

Within the NJ task force, we created roles: one member became the secretary who took minutes for all our meetings, helped to create and write the e-mail blasts to our communities, informing them and inviting them to advocate for the NJ license. Another member was the liaison for the primary sponsor of the bill. All other members maintained connection and communication with the senators and assemblymen/women where each of us lived. Yet another member created a NJ Task Force website and updated it. One member facilitated our 90-minute bi-weekly, at times weekly, planning meetings.

The dynamic of any group can go through ebbs and flows. At times the group dynamic of task force members was challenging; for example, finding a time when we could all meet was difficult due to work schedules, health issues, parenting, etc. We chose 9 p.m. for our meetings on Mondays. It was not really convenient for everyone, but it was the time the largest number of us could all meet together. We used conference calls to talk until we began using a Zoom link borrowed from the North American Drama Therapy Association (NADTA). We also canvassed all the drama therapists and dance/movement therapists in NJ and made a grid of where they lived and worked. We then created a chart that showed a list of names of the sites, type of setting, population served, and location/county where drama therapy and dance/movement therapy services were provided.

On Hill Day, the day that drama therapists and dance/movement therapists went to the state capital in Trenton to talk to legislators, we were given a room where legislators could visit to learn about our bill. Some of the task force members stayed in the room educating the legislators, and others stayed in the hallways approaching legislators. We handed out information regarding our bill along with pens that had our bill information. We put together promotional packets that educated legislators about drama therapy and dance/movement therapy along with testimony from practitioners, clients, and colleagues.

We looked at the kinds of bills the legislators supported and crafted our own communication to highlight what our profession could offer. One example was reaching out to NJ Governor Christie, who had started a task force while in office to address substance and opioid abuse. We listed all the drama therapists and dance/movement therapists working effectively with these populations in the state.

The bill had to go through the following steps:

- Both Assembly committees and Senate committees
- Regulated professions committee, NJ assembly where we gave testimony
- Assembly Floor for vote
- Senate Commerce Committee, where we gave testimony
- Senate Budget and Appropriations Committee (SBA)
- Senate Floor for vote

After the bill passed through all these steps, it went to the governor's desk. However, Governor Christie took no action on the bill before leaving office, making it necessary to start the process again with the newly elected Governor Murphy. We went through the entire process all over again.

In our testimony and advocacy before the Assembly and the Senate, we emphasized the following points that state why licensure is essential:

- Licensure will provide a means to protect consumers by ensuring that individuals calling themselves Drama Therapists and Dance/Movement Therapists have the education, clinical training, and credentialing requirements outlined in the bill.
- Licensure would improve access to drama therapy and dance/movement therapy services for NJ residents. Many organizations, such as healthcare facilities and schools, often require official "state recognition" of a credential in order to support professional services.
- Licensure would alleviate public confusion regarding the difference between professional drama therapy and dance/movement therapy services and the general use of drama and dance in healthcare and educational settings. For example, teaching artists and drama or dance teachers who are not trained in drama therapy or dance/movement therapy sometimes work with vulnerable populations like children with autism and trauma (See Laura Wood's essay in Chapter 1).

Sometimes, the legislative process does work as it was designed to, and we felt that we were well on our way to a meaningful and successful outcome. But then, there was the waiting, and waiting, and waiting – for return phone calls, e-mails, or the votes in the Assembly or Senate. Return calls never came. E-mails did not receive responses. Promises were made that the bill would be placed on the agenda for a vote, but it was not.

We worked hard, spreading the word to our supporters, urging them to contact their legislators and ask them to VOTE YES on our bill. So much work in so little time! Over and over again. And there were many times that the bill just was not voted on for reasons we often never understood.

Other challenges we faced in this tedious process included having the bill make it all the way to the governor's desk, but not be signed, causing us to start all over again in the new legislative session. There have also been numerous occasions where we tried furiously to find out who to talk to regarding what our next steps should be. It was difficult to get answers to our most pressing questions. Often, weeks and months would go by between each step along the way.

Finally, January 31, 2019, Governor Murphy conditionally vetoed the bill, meaning he would approve the bill, pending certain changes, if both houses agreed to pass the bill with the conditions. Changes were made and the bill was passed in the Assembly on November 25 and passed on December 16 in the Senate. The bill was officially approved on December 19th, 2019.

The bill did not become a law until six months after it was passed in June 2020. The next step is creating the regulatory board composed of drama therapists, dance/movement therapists, art therapists, music therapists, and recreational therapists (as the revisions provided licensure to all of these professions under the same law). This process will also take time, which is where we are now in January 2021. We are venturing into something unknown again. In a sense, we closed the "show" when the bill became a law, and now the new production is starting.

It has definitely been a learning experience for all of us. Some of our NJ Task Force team members continue to work diligently towards the establishment of the Creative Arts and Activities Therapies Board. Currently, the board has been constituted and regulations are being created. It is a long, often exhausting process, but one that we know is worth it. There are so many who will benefit from the effective services that Drama Therapists and Dance/Movement Therapists have to offer once the license is in effect.

Our task force is grateful for the support of ArtPride's Director of Advocacy & Public Policy, Ann Marie Miller. Whenever we reached out to her in need of a way to contact the community at large, Ann Marie came through for us, often immediately. She and her staff have created ways for us to reach a wider audience with our requests for contacting legislators – enhancing the effectiveness of our campaign greatly. We know we are not alone in the belief in the power of the arts to heal.

The national associations of Drama Therapy and Dance/Movement Therapy have been supportive and appreciative of the persistence and hard work that has brought the licensure process to this point. To recognize this, the American Dance Therapy Association presented the members of the NJ Task Force for Licensure of Drama Therapists and Dance/Movement Therapists with the 2017 Outstanding Achievement Award. In addition, the North American Drama Therapy Association gave a service award to this task force in 2019.

Current and Former members of NJ Task Force for Licensure of Drama Therapists and Dance/Movement Therapists: Tina Erfer, BC-DMT, LCAT, NCC; LisaGail Schwartz, MA, RDT, LCAT; Joan G. Berkowitz, LCSW, BC-DMT, NCPsyA; Brooke Campbell, MA, RDT-BCT, LCAT; Mizuho Kanazawa, LCAT, RDT-BCT; Barbara McKechnie, LPC, LCAT, RDT–BCT, TEP; Naomi Arad Broome MA BC-DMT LAC; Eri Millrod, PhD, LPC, NCC, BC-DMT; Kristin Pollock, BC-DMT, LPC, ACS.

GOING MENTAL: STOPPING STIGMA ONE STORY AT A TIME

▶ by Randy Mulder

Randy Mulder is the executive artistic director of Village Playback Theatre and co-director of the New York School of Playback Theatre.

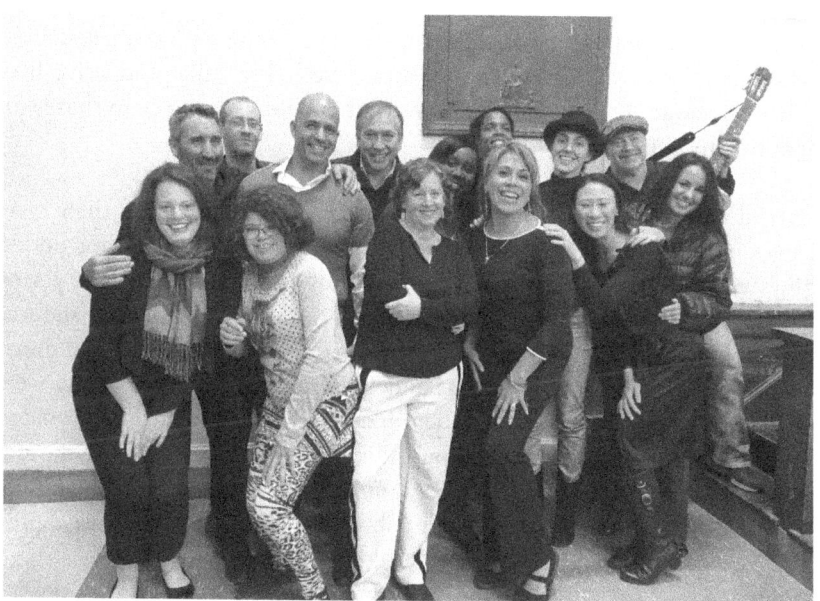

Figure 5.7 An early rehearsal with Village Playback Theatre and Citiview Connections members.

I can't remember exactly what led to my interest in applying theater to the stigma of mental illness. Was it from my experience working as clinician with patients in various psychiatric hospitals or with prisoners in the psychiatric unit at a maximum-security prison? In both places there was a blatant theme that tied them together: The patients were suffering not only from mental illness but also from the deep shame of having mental illness. I asked a prisoner, who was close to being released, how he would navigate his illness once he got out. How would he share this information with his girlfriend and his family? He looked at me with utter astonishment and said, "I'm not going to tell them. I am never going to share this information with anybody. It's not their business." His response still haunts me today.

The process of developing effective theater performances to fight mental illness stigma is complex. The decision to focus specifically on this important topic was prompted by a performance by my applied theater company, Village Playback Theatre, produced at a psycho-social clubhouse in Queens, New York.

The clubhouse's director was a former member of my company and a drama therapy colleague of mine. He invited the company to perform for the clubhouse members: adults of various ages, genders, and races who had been sidelined as a result of mental illness. Some were diagnosed at an early age and unable to continue education or seek employment. Some had graduated from college, even from Ivy League schools, and were living full, productive lives until their illness took over. In this show, we invited the audience to share stories about their mental illness.

We learned through these stories that, aside from the illness itself, there were challenges of being stigmatized. One man spoke about his family not understanding what having depression was like or how they could help. A young woman described the pain of losing her friends because they thought she was weird. Another woman was grieving over the loss of her cat who offered much companionship throughout her illness and the resulting isolation. Many were stigmatized by relatives who treated them like children or friends who avoided them. Following the show, the clubhouse director and I spoke of our mutual interest in developing some type of program to address mental health stigma. After going our separate ways, I thought about how such a collaborative program would be created and who would fund it.

There was no "aha" moment, but an idea evolved over time and was informed by work I had done in a radically different setting: Sing Sing Prison. Several years earlier, I had worked in a theater program inside Sing Sing Correctional Facility, a maximum-security prison in upstate New York. Over the course of several weeks, I taught the basics of Playback Theatre to nine prisoners.

Playback Theater is an applied theater form which is practiced internationally. Fundamentally improv-based, the audience is invited to voluntarily share stories about themselves. Often, the stories are linked to a theme chosen for the performance. The performance host, called the Conductor, selects a storyteller and informally elicits information so that the audience and performers understand the significant details of the story – when the story takes place, where, who is involved, and what happens. Then, the storyteller and audience watch as the performers enact the story (Salas, 2013; Fox, 1994).

As the prisoners gained proficiency in their Playback skills, I knew that an essential part of their learning required actually performing in front of an audience to sustain their interest. I was able to arrange a performance in the psychiatric unit within the prison. The performance was successful in three important ways. First, the prisoner audience in the psych unit attended a special new experience, at which they were invited to talk about themselves and were portrayed by people who looked, talked, acted and dressed exactly as they did. Second, the performers, also prisoners, had an unprecedented opportunity to enroll in a new identity, the theater artist, which brought them a significant sense of accomplishment and self-worth (Fox & Dauber, 1999). The final success came from the unit chief who related that it would have taken them a year or two to learn about the patients' history versus what they heard in a 10-minute story.

This performance taught me that peer-to-peer learning is invaluable. Performers on stage, who mirror the audience and share their lived experience, can connect powerfully with that audience. There is nothing comparable. It was this understanding that I brought into the collaboration between the Citiview Connections Clubhouse (Goodwill Industries of Greater New York and Northern New Jersey) and Village Playback Theatre.

The Project

The goal of the project was to reduce the stigma of mental health by providing Playback performances throughout the borough of Queens, New York City. The performances would allow people with mental illness to talk openly about the challenges and triumphs of living with their disease with the explicit intention to normalize the illness and their lives. With the help of Russ Roten, the Citiview Connections Clubhouse director, we identified our audience: Agencies and organizations that provide services to people with mental illness. Another secondary, but equally important goal was to educate the family and friends of those with the illness and the general public about ways we can increase our awareness around stigma and what actions we can take to decrease it.

The performers were professional artists who were members of Village Playback Theatre and selected members of the Clubhouse. These members, later known as "Citiview Artists," were adults who had chronic and persistent mental illness and were interested in learning Playback Theatre and participating in this project on decreasing stigma.

One critical step before launching the project was finding funding. This is always a challenge. I went straight to the top and applied for a federally funded grant bestowed by the National Endowment of the Arts (NEA). The application itself was daunting. Vast amounts of information were required: Narrative descriptions, budgets, financial projections, video and photographs of past performances. However, what we were proposing seemed precisely the kind of project the prestigious NEA was looking to fund. We were thrilled to receive the grant! Now we could reserve performance venues and pay the many people involved in the productions.

The auditioning of Citiview Artists centered on a number of factors: Interest in the project, availability, maturity, self-awareness, integrity, and the desire to exercise spontaneity and creativity (Nachmanovitch, 1990). As a clinician, I was aware that there can be many factors that can decrease one's ability to be spontaneous and creative, including the types and dosages of medication, general mood, and other stressors. The other two factors I considered were the ability to get along with other people and to follow directions. These may seem like basic and non-remarkable characteristics. Everybody has good days and bad days. But, when dealing with mental illness, good and bad days can have more weight and be more difficult to manage.

This first audition was focused on play: To see how freely people participated, the degree to which they could understand and follow rules, and their interaction between one another. They were wonderful. Playful, laughing, joking with one another. Some were more talkative, while others were more subdued. The second time we met, interested Clubhouse members brought a completed questionnaire that indicated any experience in the theater or the performing arts, any prior commitments, and a statement about why they were interested in this project. Many were very articulate and showed a great deal of enthusiasm. A few had prepared resumes which accompanied their completed forms. It was difficult making choices. We ultimately invited six Clubhouse members to join Village Playback Theatre actors.

Our early rehearsals were focused on getting Citiview Artists comfortable with one another and teaching the basic foundations of Playback Theatre. We told

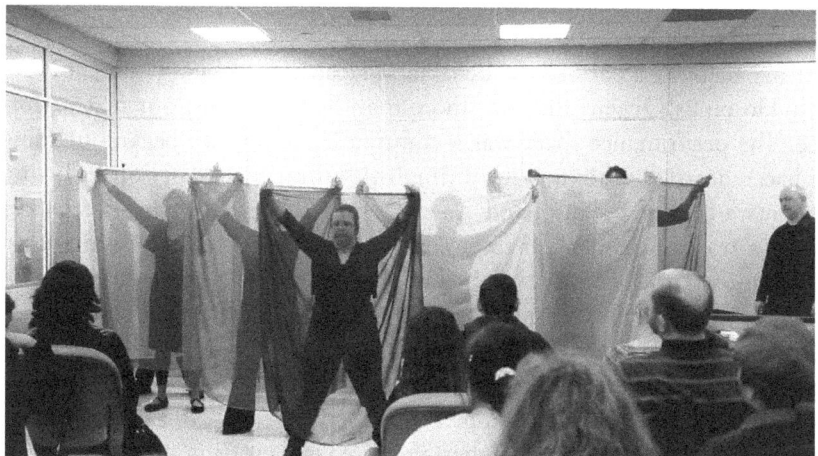

Figure 5.8 The opening of our first show at Queens Hospital.

stories about ourselves. As rehearsals progressed, the stories became more inti-
mate, dotted with personal events and references to experiences that were sel-
dom shared. At the same time, I was busy plotting out where we'd perform and
on what dates.

Identifying each person's performative strengths was a part of the devising of
our shows. Some were more physically expressive and able to use their bodies
to express feelings and mood. Others were strong vocally and were more at
ease expressing themselves with words. All these attributes were considered as
we started to figure out how we would integrate these new performers into our
existing cast and what talents to amplify. We had to keep in mind that we had
people who had no theater experience, had never stood in front of a large group
of people under the direction of a director working in conjunction with other
performers, much less stood under a stage light and shared something personal
about themselves.

I knew that we needed to spread out the performances, so we had time between
shows to reconvene and process what had happened, the impact it had on the
performers, and the effect on the audience. I often take the approach that the
best way to prepare for a performance is to perform in a performance. That logic
may sound like a contradiction. It is not. At some point you have to acknowledge that the artists' performance is not going to improve with more rehearsal.
The only thing that will accomplish that is to get in front of an audience. After
putting in months of rehearsal, it was show time.

Opening Performances

With Russ' help, we identified the Behavioral Health Treatment Center at NYC Health+Hospitals Queens that was more than happy to host our first performance. The performance space was a community room. We began our show as we had rehearsed. After making a ritualistic entrance, one person following the other, we created a tableau and, on cue, everybody raised their sheer pieces of fabric in front of them. In effect, we were shielding ourselves or veiling ourselves from the audience while at the same time being seen by them and able to see them. One by one, we spoke behind the fabric sharing something about ourselves in relationship to mental illness, the theme of our performance. A few moments after everyone had finished their introductions, one by one we dropped our fabric pieces and stepped over them, symbolizing that whatever we were fearing or hiding from earlier, now we were crossing over this barrier into a new threshold (Queens Councils for the Arts, 2016). The visual was eye-catching. The audience responded immediately.

People shared experiences about their day, and then about the people in their lives. One woman shared that she was being mistreated by her caregiver, and she was afraid to be with her. The story of abuse and neglect invited another woman to share experiences of her childhood when she was sexually abused by relatives, neglected, and often hungry. These were tender stories about heroic people who had dealt with so much trauma and survived it.

Many of our audience members were very enthusiastic about the show and were eager to talk to us. A few doctors on the psychiatric staff invited me to their offices to speak privately. They were warm and generous and expressed gratitude for our show and its unique and much needed place among psychiatric care. We left feeling buoyed. This was exactly the kind of experience we needed to build our confidence and provide us momentum to continue the other performances which lay ahead.

Managing nervousness is a key part of my job. The second show was a few weeks later at Citiview. Here, the Citiview Artists would be performing in front of their peers and staff of the Clubhouse. My approach was to provide as much practice time as possible so that the performers gained mastery of the skills needed to perform by exercising those skills over and over again until they became second nature. In turn, the sense of mastery built confidence. We achieved this and the show went without a hitch. For our third performance we returned to the Behavior Health Treatment Center to another section of the psychiatric unit. As with our first show, people were responsive.

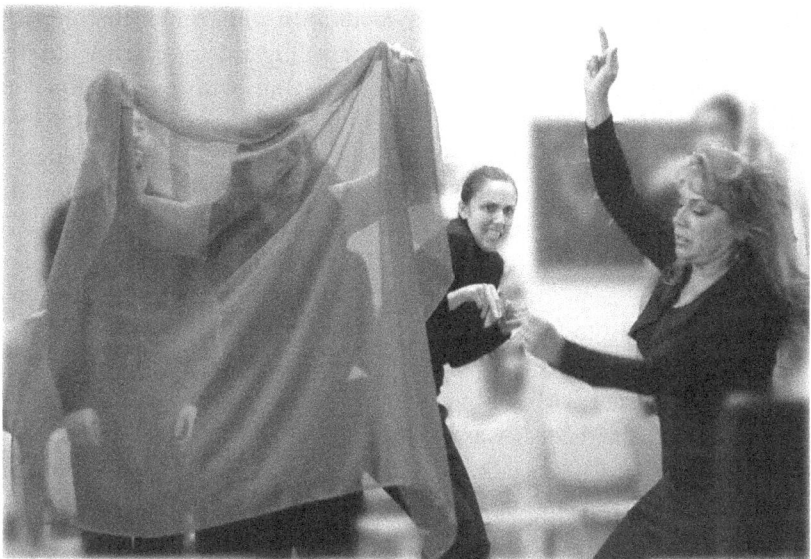

Figure 5.9 Artists playing back a story at Citiview Connections Clubhouse.

Public Performances

The shows that were the most complex to produce and had the largest audiences were our public shows held at the historic Queens Theatre. Unlike the spaces in which we performed our private shows, this theater had a legit stage with stage lighting and raked seating for the audience. These performances were also different from all the other shows because our focus was to educate the general public about mental illness and the stigma attached to it. We had to devise different material that would achieve this goal.

We knew that the audiences at the Queens Theatre may not have had any direct relationship to mental illness, so we would need to amplify moments where they could learn what this illness was about. Our introductions spoke directly to this. One performer's introduction began, "My mom was a single mom who suffered from crippling anxiety." Another shared, "After the death of my mother, I was hospitalized four times in a psychiatric ward... I thought I would never get out." A third performer described her depression by revealing, "It's frustrating and disheartening that my family and friends think that taking a shower or brushing your teeth every day is easy. It isn't for me."

Mental illness does not discriminate with respect to age, race, gender, education, socio-economic status, and other factors. In our combined company, it was not only Citiview Artists who were managing this disease. A number of Village Playback actors were either directly dealing with mental illness or had family members who had mental illnesses. From these shared identities, I invited a handful of them to write monologues describing their experience. They gladly participated, and I interspersed these monologues throughout the show. These autobiographical speeches served as invitations for the audience to discover from the performers themselves what the illness looked and felt like. They also functioned as prompts for people in the audience who had personal and direct relationships to mental illness.

One monologue started with, "My mom and I were very close... I lost my identity the second she died. It was like, where am I? Who am I? What am I doing?... I thought the TV was talking to me. I thought the radio was telling me that I was winning prizes" (Village Playback Theatre, 2019).

The success of the integration of our Citiview Artists and the performances rested largely on the shoulders of the Village Playback Theatre performers. They were consistently warm and supportive of these new artists. They answered their questions and applauded gleefully when a new skill was learned. Their expertise as experienced performers functioned as a container for all the tensions, and the use of their craft – their ability to create spontaneous and creative moments – was moving not only to the audience but inspiring to the artists onstage (Rowe, 2007).

The stories shared by audience members during these three public performances were touching, harrowing, courageous, and inspiring. On our first night, representatives from the NYC Department of Mental Health and Hygiene attended. A woman from that office graciously and generously shared her own experience with the illness. The adult children of one of our Citiview Artists shared that they had never before understood what their mother was talking about or the extent of the suffering that she had endured. With tears in their eyes and in quiet voices, they said now they understood. A widow shared lovingly about her husband who, after suffering for several years with mental illness, had committed suicide. She bravely educated all of us not to demonize him or his actions. One woman spoke of her struggles with homelessness and another of coming to terms with her schizophrenia diagnosis.

These stories were firsthand accounts from people who were suffering and surviving the throes of mental illness. Learning about mental illness in print,

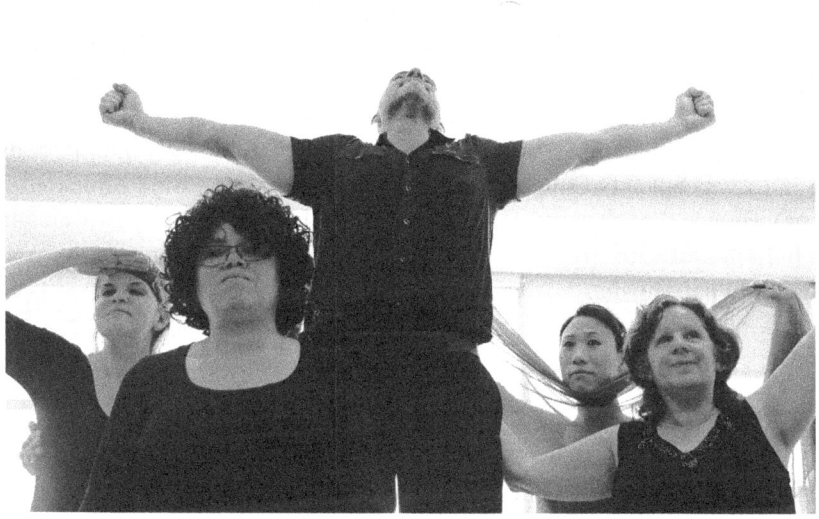

Figure 5.10 Our third show, another performance on a different unit at Queens Hospital.

on screen, or through a podcast, does not compare to the energetically connected experience of the stage. This was confirmed by surveys sent to all the attendees; their responses were unanimous. These performances helped educate audiences and diminished mental health stigma. Another teaching tool, available several months later, was a short video which chronicled three weeks of rehearsal leading up to and including the public performances (Village Playback Theatre, 2019).

Final Performances

We gave two additional performances following the Queens Theatre shows. One was for queer and trans adults with mental illness and the other for men living in a veterans' homeless shelter. At this last performance, I noticed a gentleman loudly talking to himself. Once the show began, his self-talk became louder, and I decided to give him my full attention; I asked him if he wanted to join us and tell a story. He hesitated for a second or two, nodded, and joined us by sitting next to me. He introduced himself as "Clarence." Rather than sharing a story, Clarence asked, "Can we sing the Battle Hymn of the Republic?" I quickly looked over to our musician, and he motioned he was ready. "Great, why don't we all sing it!" I replied. We jumped into the song, and when we arrived at the chorus, the song became familiar to most people in the room, and the music section swelled. To my surprise, Clarence launched into a sweet harmony line that I hadn't heard before but fit perfectly with the melody. After the second verse, we closed with a rousing "Glory, glory hallelujah. His truth is marching on." When we finished, the energy in the room had completely changed, including Clarence's entire demeanor. I glanced quickly into the audience and saw people's faces light up with smiles, but no expression compared to that of Clarence. For that moment, his mind, his body, and his spirit were one with himself and with us. Sometimes the lifting of the stigma results from an invitation to participate.

Closing Thoughts

From the beginning, one of our key goals for the Citiview Artists was for them to have a successful experience – that they not be put in a position of committing themselves to a goal that was outside of their reach. We wanted them to have a process, much like running a marathon, which takes considerable training and where there would be good days and bad days, yet once the race began, and as they continued pacing themselves, placing one foot in front of the other, they would reach the finish line.

A more explicit goal was to banish the secrecy in talking about mental health and normalize the topic. For audiences who had the illness we wanted them to identify with the performers, many of whom themselves were in recovery. That maybe they could get to the point one day where they could approach their friends and neighbors and say, "I have a mental illness, so what?" We hoped that they would be able to stretch themselves and take risks to do things that they didn't think were possible.

Finally, we wanted to educate people who didn't have much direct connection to this disease to see what it looked and felt liked, to increase their understanding and their empathy. All of these goals were achieved. To continue the metaphor, I recognized that it was not only the trainees who benefited from participating in this race, but my seasoned performers and I were educated and inspired by the audiences we performed for, and especially by the Citiview Artists. These artists, with their determination, courage, generosity, and resilience, carried us along with them across that finish line, for which we are forever grateful.

References

Fox, J. (1994). *Acts of service: Spontaneity, commitment, tradition in the nonscripted theatre.* Tusitala Publishing.

Fox, J., & Dauber, H. (Eds.). (1999). *Gathering voices: Essays on playback theatre.* Tusitala Publishing.

Nachmanovitch, S. (1990). *Free play: Improvisation in life and art.* Tarcher/Putnam.

Queens Council for the Arts. (2016, May 17). Meet QAF awardee goodwill industries & village playback theatre [Blog]. Retrieved from https://www.queenscouncilarts.org/blog/2016/5/17/meet-qaf-awardee-goodwill-industries-village-playback-theatre

Rowe, N. (2007). *Playing the other: Dramatizing personal narratives in playback theatre.* Jessica Kingsley Publishers.

Salas, J. (2013). *Improvising real life: Personal story in playback theatre.* (4th ed.). Tusitala Publishing.

Village Playback Theatre. (2019, March 12). VPT's going mental: Stopping mental health stigma one story at a time [Video]. YouTube. Retrieved from https://www.youtube.com/watch?v=Ldvhg6rMYXs&feature=youtu.be

INDEX

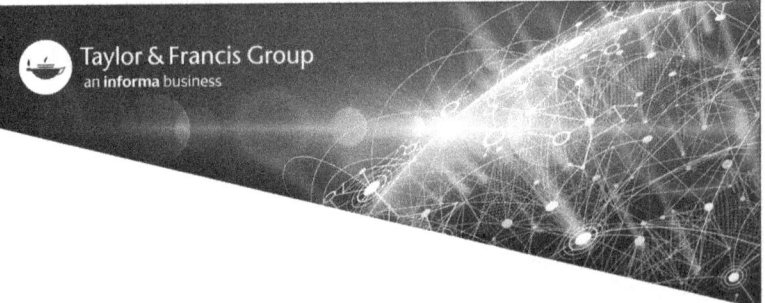
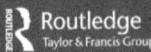
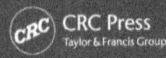